Breathing

Space

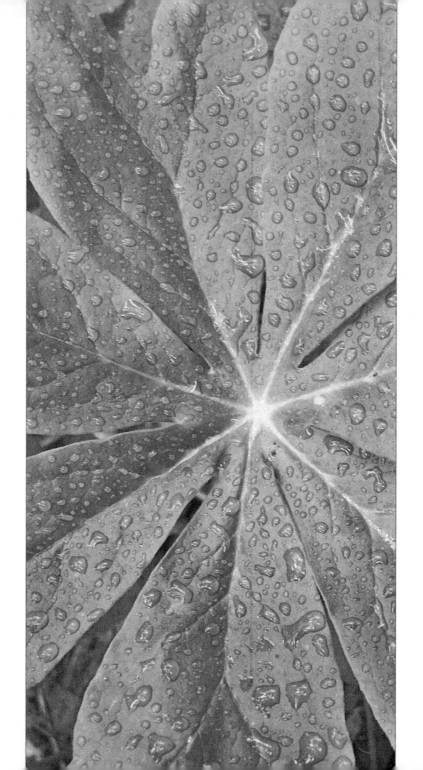

Breathing Space

TWELVE LESSONS
FOR THE MODERN WOMAN

Katrina Repka
and Alan Finger

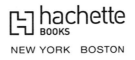

NEW YORK BOSTON

Hachette Books
Hachette Book Group
1290 Avenue of the Americas
New York, NY 10104

www.HachetteBookGroup.com

Originally published by Hyperion.
First Hachette Books edition: September 2014

Hachette Books is a division of Hachette Book Group, Inc.
The Hachette Books name and logo are trademarks of Hachette Book Group, Inc.

The publisher is not responsible for websites (or their content) that are not owned by the publisher.

Library of Congress Cataloging-in-Publication Data
Repka, Katrina.
    Breathing space : twelve lessons for the modern woman / Katrina
Repka and Alan Finger.
        p. cm.
    ISBN-13: 978-1-4013-0347-1
    1. Breathing exercises. 2. Hatha yoga. I. Finger, Alan, 1946– II. Title.
    RA782.R47   2008
    613'.192—dc22
                                                    2008037982

Design by Fearn Cutler de Vicq

To Ferb, with love and gratitude

Contents

Acknowledgments

Without the following people this book would not have been born, survived infancy, or grown to maturity:

Chris Grey
Jennifer Lyons
Ayesha Pande
Jill Parsons-Stern
Ellen Archer
Pam Dorman
Sarah Landis
The team at Voice
Mom
Dad
The ISHTA Yoga community
. . . and Alan, of course

THANK YOU!

A Message from Katrina

⸺

This is the story of a year I spent in New York, studying with Yoga Master Alan Finger.

It turned out to be such a life-changing experience for me that I wanted to share with other women what I had learned from him and help them to make the same kinds of important discoveries about themselves that I did.

When I met Alan, I lacked confidence and was prone to self-criticism and emotional fluctuations. I could not let go of the past—and I was afraid of the future. To be honest, I did not know who I was or where I was going. Thanks to his knowledge and guidance, the time I spent with Alan has been transformative. I am more decisive and assured now. I have become more like the person I always wanted to be.

If you have ever wondered whether you are the person you really want to be, or felt at all hindered by personal obstacles and uncertain of your true role in life (even if you are successful in your career or chosen field, or perhaps *because of* this success), our book will help you to remove the emotional blocks and mental traps that are delaying your progress.

In twelve simple, clear exercises we show you how you can use the power of your own breath to discover who you are and what you want. These exercises are designed to purge anxiety and negativity, and to clear and cleanse the body and mind so that you can make your own decisions about the life you want to live. By harnessing the breath to unite your body, mind, and spirit, you will learn to move forward confidently on the path that you choose.

Alan was guiding me as I learned the exercises in this book. You may find it helpful to record yourself reading an exercise aloud and then play it back as you practice (remember to leave a suitable length of silence where the instructions indicate passing time), or share the exercise with a friend and take turns leading each other; do whatever helps you to relax and enjoy the experience with the least effort.

I also benefited from writing down what I felt before, during, and after each exercise. This became a record of my feelings as the breath began to work its magic in my life.

The breathing exercises in this book are gentle and safe, but if you have a preexisting medical condition, please check with your doctor before doing them. Pregnant women should *not* hold the breath, although, of course, breathing in and out is highly recommended! (For detailed instructions, please refer to individual exercises.)

Breath work is one aspect of a full yogic practice; there is much, much more to learn, if you are interested. The first step is finding a good local teacher—someone experienced who can guide you (an international listing of teachers trained by Alan can be found on his website www.ishtayoga.com). There are many different styles of yoga; whichever you choose, do look for a certified instructor, someone you feel comfortable with. Remember always to listen to your body and your breath, and never to overdo things.

This is a true story, but the order of some events has been changed, and my conversations with Alan and others are not always recounted *exactly* as they happened. Nonetheless, the substance of everything we discuss in the book is real and true. Also, except for Alan's, the names of all of the characters (and a few of the places) have been changed. As for the breaths, some of them have Sanskrit names that we have replaced with English ones to make them more accessible.

So let's begin.

Namaste. Which in Sanskrit means "The light in me bows to the light in you."

Katrina

Breathing

Space

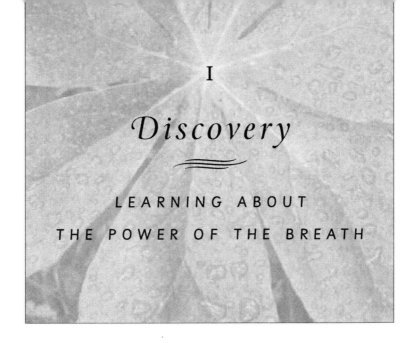

I

Discovery

LEARNING ABOUT THE POWER OF THE BREATH

What am I doing with my life?

The old, familiar question. The one I thought I'd left behind.

I slouched in the hard plastic chair and stared at the sudsy laundry tumbling in the washer across from me. Around and around it went one way. Then around and around the other. Nine o'clock on a Thursday night in New York City. I should have been out on the town. Instead, I was sitting in my apartment building's basement laundry room. Getting ready to use the dryer. Fold the laundry. And find my boyfriend's missing sock. Although I had no objection to the title Domestic Goddess, it wasn't at the top of my list. Nor was it the role I'd had in mind when I arrived in New York four months ago, intent on a voyage of self-discovery.

———

My life in Manhattan was supposed to be the complete opposite of my life in Calgary, Alberta. I would be thinner, smarter, happier, hipper. My work would be glamorous, my days and nights filled with excitement and fascinating new friends. I wasn't going to settle for the comfortable routine that had threatened to stifle me in my old hometown.

To live in New York had been my dream since childhood. When I was only three, I asked my father if we could go and live there—I must have seen the city in a film and been impressed by the skyscrapers—and he tried to dissuade me by saying that it was a dirty, scary place. But then he said pretty much the same thing about the Chinook Centre mall in southwest Calgary. Some twenty-five years later, I had my chance. In the summer of 2000, I persuaded the University of Calgary, where I was studying for a master's degree in communications, to let me fulfill part of the course requirements by taking classes at The New School in Greenwich Village.

Before I left for New York, I had broken off the relationship with my longtime boyfriend, David. My friends thought I was crazy; he had a house in a new suburban development, a Jeep Cherokee, and money in mutual funds—everything a Calgary girl could want. But when he asked me to marry him, I turned him down. They all said he was the ideal husband, but I was far from ready to be the ideal wife—someone like my mother, who, while she was married to my father, had waited on him hand and foot.

Some two weeks into my New York study trip, I was in The New School computer lab, where I had taken to going during my lunch break to write up class notes and check my emails, when I heard someone behind me say: "Is this funny? I need someone to tell me if it is, before I hand it in."

The voice was British. It was a nice voice. I turned around. It appeared that the fellow was talking to me.

"Would you?" he said. "You look like someone who might give me an honest answer."

He was older than most of the students: late thirties, at a guess. And better dressed. He wore Paul Smith glasses, and his head was shaved. It was a well-shaped head. Coming from Calgary, however, I thought that someone who looked as cool as this had to be gay.

"Sure," I said.

He handed it to me. I read the piece. It was funny, and I laughed.

"You're not doing that just to be nice, are you?" he said.

"No, it's good. Really."

"I'm never very sure," he said. "Thanks."

"Are you a teacher or student?"

His name was Matthew, he was from London, and he'd come to New York to pursue a master's degree in creative writing.

A few days later I was back in the lab, and Matthew was there again, too. This time he asked me out to dinner. *Why not?* I thought. He was witty, he was stylish, and I was currently short of dinner invitations.

He took me to a swanky restaurant just off Gramercy Park. It was a warm evening and we sat outside in the garden. There was candlelight. A crisp white wine. And a full moon. I looked around at the other couples seated nearby. It was all very romantic. Just my luck to be stuck with the charming gay guy. But the more we talked, the more I began to doubt my first impression. We were finishing the bottle when I plucked up the courage to ask.

"You are gay, right?"

He burst out laughing.

Our romance was intense, and made all the more so because in only six weeks I'd have to cut short the great time I was having and return home. I wasn't excited about the prospect. My job as regional marketing manager for a wireless phone company was uninspiring, my best friends were all getting married and having babies (and waiting to hear when I would), and my mother was still expecting me to explain why I'd broken off my relationship with David. As for my father, all he would want to hear about my summer sojourn was that I'd finally gotten the whole big-city thing out of my system and was ready to settle down to a long, steady career, just as he had.

To my delight, Matthew and I kept our relationship going after I left New York. I found excuses to return. He visited Canada. We traveled to London, where I was introduced to his friends and family. We ran up phone bills, logged hours at our computers emailing, and soon realized that what we had together was stronger than just a summer fling. Matthew had been in the travel business before moving to New York to go back to school with the intention of becoming a writer; I admired his desire to reinvent himself, as well as his openness and generosity. He told me I made him laugh. Even so, neither of us made any promises for the future.

Yet Matthew was the first person I called when, a few months after my return home, I was summoned into my boss's office and told I was being downsized. (How true—by the time I left her office I felt about two inches tall.)

"Come back to New York," he said, when I called with the news. "You can live with me and find out who you really are and what you want to do with your life."

With my job gone, I had no reason to stay in Calgary. I had every reason to go to New York. It took me about five seconds to say yes.

As soon as I had hung up the phone, I began to have second thoughts. This is a family trait, having second thoughts. We can't even go out to dinner together without having half a dozen options and then debating the pros and cons of each until we have exhausted ourselves. I lay in bed that night and listed my options:

1. Stay in Calgary and do nothing (safe, reassuring, predictable)
2. Stay in Calgary and change my life completely (Q: How does one do that in a city where the weather is the main topic of conversation?)
3. Go to New York and start a new life (doing what? How?)

Option 3 was obviously the most inviting, but also the most terrifying. By morning I had made my decision. I phoned my father to tell him the news and ask for his blessing.

"Are you planning to get married?" were his first words.

"That's not relevant at the moment, Dad," I said. "We want to live together and see how it goes."

"And if it goes wrong?"

"I'll worry about that if it does."

"That's not what I call good planning."

"Dad, this isn't a business venture."

"No? And how are you going to finance this alternative lifestyle?"

"I thought I'd do a little drug dealing on the side."

Silence.

"Dad, Matthew said that he would support me until I figure out what I want to do."

"Oh, yes? And you trust him to do the right thing?"

"Absolutely," I said, crossing my fingers.

"I don't get it," he said. "Everybody wants to come and live in Calgary—it's the fastest-growing, best-value midwestern city in North America—and you want to leave!"

I can always come back, I almost said. But stopped myself.

I didn't need Dad's blessing, after all. Just talking to him had convinced me that I was doing the right thing. Secretly, I think, he admired my courage, although he'd never have said so to my face. He once admitted to me that he had always wanted to be a writer. But following *his* father's wishes, he had stuck with corporate law for thirty-five years. I didn't want my life to turn into a list of things I only wished I had done.

When I told my mother, she was silent. And since she is a great talker, that meant she wasn't convinced. Why would I want to leave, she was surely thinking, when I had everything anyone could ever want—friends, family, career—at home? But it just wasn't the life I wanted. I tried to explain, but I could tell that she was hurt. She had devoted her life to her family and wanted to keep us together. And now I was running off.

It had been tough, but I had told my parents. The hard part was done. The next day I bought my ticket.

————

I arrived in August, and Matthew and I spent the rest of the summer relaxing and enjoying the city. In the autumn, Matthew was starting his degree, and I would be teaching marketing and advertising at the Fashion Institute of Technology (FIT), a job one of my classmates at The New School the previous summer had helped to arrange. I also signed up for far too many evening classes—poetry, cooking, painting, and sculpture—in a mad rush to try to become the kind of person I had always wanted to be. The kind of person I saw all around me: a cultivated, cultured New Yorker who had it together, inside and out.

I was just finding my feet when, a few weeks later, the planes struck the World Trade Center. I panicked. The sleepy safety of Calgary had never looked so appealing. I thought seriously about going home, but by the time flights had been restored, I knew that if I gave in to my fears and did go, it was unlikely I would ever leave again; it would be too easy to get sucked back into my old, comfortable way of life. Besides, my pride wouldn't let me. If I backed down now, it would be as if I had never left in the first place.

But everything I had once enjoyed doing now made me anxious. Wandering the streets, watching the bustle and flow of city life, sitting at a café—I may have looked carefree, but I was on my guard all the time. I couldn't ride the subway without eyeing the other passengers as if one of them might be carrying a bomb. Didn't that big guy over there in the bulging suit look suspicious? What about those kids with their thirty-pound backpacks? Or the lady clutching the explosive miniature poodle?

I tried to take my mind off my worries by concentrating on my work at FIT and doing regular yoga classes. In what I now mentally referred to as "my old life," I'd always found a physical satisfaction in how the vigorous form of yoga—Ashtanga—had stretched and strengthened my muscles and left me feeling calm and relaxed.

I had started doing Ashtanga a couple of years before, because I was told it would complement the running and skiing I loved so much; at my regular Calgary studio, I knew the workout and was friendly with many of the students and teachers. But now, in New York, I could not find a yoga studio where I felt at home. To tell the truth, I was intimidated by all of them. Every class I signed up for was full of gorgeous, thin females in fashionable outfits who just had to be models or actresses. I was in awe of these BlackBerry-toting, Nuala-wearing creatures, who practiced to perfection. I could only begin to imagine how fabulous their lives were. The parties they went to. The clubs they hung out at. The laundry room I sat in.

At the same time, I was put off by the thought of those teachers who had been recommended to me as old-school yogis. I remembered only too well the old-school yogi I had gone to in Nepal (while I was a volunteer with the Kathmandu Environmental Education Project in my early twenties), where I had been the sole Westerner (and woman) in a group of rail-thin men in lungis, who spent most of their time chanting, doing obscure breathing exercises, and trying to levitate.

When I arrived in New York, I'd been practicing yoga for nearly seven years, but next to the locals I felt unstylish and out of place. So I stopped. For the next few months I taught my class at FIT, came home, had dinner, and went to bed. Gradually the anxiety that I felt in the wake of 9/11 gave way to apathy. My new life just wasn't what I had hoped for. I went out less and less. I became dispirited.

Here I was in the city of my dreams with a man I thought I loved—and instead of finding myself, I was as lost as I'd ever been.

———

I shoved another wet load of laundry into the dryer, fed it some quarters, and fell back into the plastic chair. I didn't want to return to the apartment, where Matthew was no doubt watching his favorite film, *Barton Fink*, for the millionth time. Why he loved it so much was beyond me. Whenever I sat down to watch it with him, I found my mind wandering. Then I felt disappointed with myself that I couldn't share his enthusiasm and began to agonize over whether this meant we had some fundamental incompatibility. Or whether I was just stupid.

To stop these thoughts, I gave in to my guilty pleasure: working my way through the discarded copies of *People* and *Us Weekly* that were neatly stacked on the laundry room table. Then I moved on to *Elle*, but the photos of impossibly thin, impossibly beautiful women only depressed me. With fifteen minutes still left on the dryer cycle, I picked up a copy of *New York* magazine and began to read a piece about the top yoga studios in the city. I was about to pass on to the next article when I came across a photograph of a man dressed all in white, facing the camera, calmly balancing on one leg. His eyes seemed to be looking into me.

I scrutinized the accompanying text. He was, it said, one of the most respected of all yogis living in the West. His name was Alan Finger. There was something about him that I found reassuring, even compelling. I stood up, clutching the magazine. I knew what I had to do.

———

The following afternoon I took the subway to Broadway and Twenty-third. A cold wind raked the back of my neck and slipped down the collar of my coat as I hurried toward Nineteenth Street. It was almost Christmas, and Fifth Avenue was clogged with a rush of last-minute holiday shoppers. The traffic was bumper-to-bumper, horns blasting. I finally located the building where the yoga studio was and took the elevator to the fourth floor. When the doors opened, I was greeted with warm air, incense, soft lighting, and the sounds of tinkling water and subdued voices. I felt a wave of positive energy flowing over me. *This* was what I had been looking for. I went up to the reception desk and asked if I could take Alan's class.

"Have you been to one of his classes before?" the pretty, dark-haired girl asked.

"No, I'm new," I said. "Not to yoga, but to Alan. I'm Katrina."

"Hey. I'm Charlie. Would you take this clipboard and fill out the form for me? Just the usual stuff: name, address, star sign—"

"Aha! A new student, I believe."

I turned around—and found myself face-to-face with a not very tall, slightly overweight man decked out in a trim gray beard, white shirt, and jeans. Was this *the* Alan Finger? He was so friendly and . . . normal-looking. From my powerful reaction to the magazine photo, I had expected him to radiate some otherworldly magnetism; instead I had to suppress the thought that he bore a more than passing resemblance to a gigantic garden gnome.

"Or perhaps," Alan continued, "she has come to read the meter?" He pointed at the clipboard.

Charlie let out a high-pitched laugh. "Alan," she said, "this is Katrina."

He nodded. "*Namaste.* Now please excuse me: class is starting in a few minutes and I must prepare myself. Charlie, would you do me a big favor and send down for a Venti nonfat chai latte, extra hot? And whatever you would like for yourself. I'll see you in class, Katrina."

Charlie handed him a bundle of letters and papers. He opened the door to a small adjoining room and went inside.

Right away I was drawn to Alan's joviality and intrigued by the idea that he drank chai lattes. My teacher in Canada—a hippie who called himself Wonderwing—had been adamant that spiritual realization required you to abstain from sugar, caffeine, and all forms of commercialism.

I finished filling out the form, handed the clipboard to Charlie, and followed her to the studio.

The large room was packed with sixty or so students of all shapes, sizes, and ages; this was very different from the other classes I'd been to, and I immediately felt at home. Some people were chatting together animatedly, others were sitting cross-legged in meditation or lying on their backs with their eyes closed. I unrolled my mat at the back of the class and sat down to wait. After a few minutes, Alan entered and walked toward the podium at the front of the room, greeting people right and left.

He sat down in a cross-legged position. "Let us begin," he said. "We have a new student today: Katrina. Welcome!"

A few students turned to me and smiled. I smiled back, even though it made me feel self-conscious to be singled out.

"We travel a long distance in our lives," Alan began, "and must search in many directions before we find the true path. We may ask for help along the way, but in the end only we know what is right for us, only we can make the decisions that will lead us to discover our true selves."

I felt that he was looking directly at me.

"We all possess a powerful guide on our journey to the truth. It's given to us at birth, and yet most of us are entirely unaware of it—the breath. The yogis consider the breath to be one of our most precious personal assets, the key to unlocking the inner self. But we're so filled with tension and stress that many of us are physically unable to take a full, deep breath. Instead of unlocking the inner self, we confine it."

I realized that I was in fact holding my breath and let it out as inconspicuously as I could.

Alan explained that when a baby is born, it takes full, deep, natural breaths. Then, as we grow older, the body acquires certain unhealthy habits in order to deal with the many demands that life makes on us. We hunch our shoulders and round our backs while we work on the computer. We spend so much time in cars that we shuffle instead of taking long strides when we walk. Our necks are stiff because we think too much, and our chests are tight because we are full of pent-up emotion. Result? We can no longer take in a full breath. Our bodies are all bound up inside.

"It's like wearing a jacket that's too tight," Alan said. "You simply cannot move freely. You have no space. No room. *You become a prisoner inside yourself.*"

Outside, an emergency vehicle started up its siren, and I was instantly on guard. Alan stopped speaking and looked out of the window. When the commotion had died down, he turned back to us and said: "We cannot change what will happen in the world outside. We can only change our-selves."

Alan's words were already making so much sense to me. I had hoped that just by moving to New York I would feel different. But the truth was, I didn't. I had been trying to change everything on the outside, but perhaps the answers were to be found elsewhere.

"Freeing the breath is the first step toward creating the space in the body necessary to release your true self," Alan said. "Properly applied, the breath will help you to regain the energy and exuberance you had as a small child, when time had no meaning and the future was full of promise. Once you free the body, you can free the mind, which leads you upward to the spirit. From the body, to the mind, to the spirit. Three parts that unite through the breath to become one whole."

Alan then asked us to lie down on the floor, close our eyes, and begin to breathe in and out through the nose.

"Please draw your awareness to the breath," he said. "Without judging it in any way—whether it's right or wrong, good or bad—notice how the breath is moving in your body."

My breathing was rapid and shallow at first, but as I re-laxed, it slowed down and deepened. I was falling into a dreamlike state when his voice called me to attention.

"Where does your breath begin and end?"

With my mouth closed, my breath entered through the nostrils, touched the back of the throat, and then passed downward until it came to rest in my belly.

"Now imagine the pattern your breath makes as it enters and leaves."

Pattern? That was a hard one. I felt that my breath was coming and going in all directions, like leaves in a high wind.

What kind of pattern was it *supposed* to make? I was starting to feel lost.

Then Alan said, "Don't force it. Don't tighten up. Just relax and study your breathing. Is it smooth and even? Short and choppy? Deep or shallow? Hard or soft? Give voice to whatever thoughts come into your head."

Fuzzy, I thought, and *violet, animal, fresh, accordion, Vivaldi . . . life.*

Then my mind went sort of blank, and when I was next conscious of thinking, it was about what to have for dinner— pizza? Or salad? It would have to be salad. I was having one of my fat days.

"Don't worry if your mind wanders," Alan said. "Just gently draw your awareness back to the breath."

His voice helped me to find my focus again.

"Now, place one hand on your belly and one hand on your chest. Notice the hand on your chest. Do you feel it rising as you breathe in? Does your rib cage also flare out to the sides? Do you feel any movement in your upper back as you breathe?"

My chest and back weren't moving much, so I tried to draw in more air. This gave me the uncomfortable sensation that I was about to burst. I had to stop for a moment.

"Bring your awareness to your belly. As you breathe in, do you feel the front of your abdomen lifting? Do you feel the breath causing movement in your lower back? What about your pelvic floor, can you feel it moving with your breath?"

My belly seemed to be moving much more than my chest, and I could feel my lower back expanding slightly as I breathed in. There was even some movement in my pelvic floor.

"Now, on the exhalation, feel your belly drawing back toward your spine and your pelvic floor drawing in and up."

That was harder.

"Keep your eyes closed," he said, "and take a minute for your breath to adjust. Then, when you're ready, roll over onto your right side and slowly come back up to a seated position."

For the next hour, Alan led us through a sequence of yoga postures and a seated meditation. When the class ended, I made my way to the front. Everything was glowing, inside and out.

"Thank you, Alan," I said. "I feel great." And it was true: the tension and anxiety that had oppressed me for weeks were suddenly gone.

"That's the feeling of yoga," Alan said. "Practice the breath discovery exercise every day for two weeks to become aware of your breathing patterns. Then please come and see me and tell me how you're feeling."

In all my years of doing yoga, this was the first time I had truly appreciated the power of the breath, and I left the studio full of anticipation. This *was* what I had been looking for. I was confident that with Alan's help I would begin to find the answers to my many questions. And more. I was determined to practice the breathing exercise and then return to see him. I didn't want to get too excited—I often do and then am disappointed when something doesn't measure up to my expectations—but, after all, what did I have to lose?

Breath Focus 1: DISCOVERY

Time: 10–15 minutes

Props (optional): bolster, pillow, or eye pad

1. Find a quiet place, free from distraction.

2. Lie down on your back. If your lower back feels sensitive, bend your knees (you can place them over a bolster or pillow, if you have one handy).

3. Close your eyes and, if you like, place an eye pad over them.

4. Start to breathe in and out through your nose, becoming aware of your breath. Without judging it in any way, notice how the breath moves in your body. Where does it begin and end? Is it fast or slow? What pattern does it make as it enters and leaves?

5. Notice the composition of your breath. Is it smooth and even? Short and choppy? Deep or shallow? Hard or soft? When you inhale, does your torso expand or contract? What happens when you exhale?

6. If you become aware at any point that your mind has wandered, gently draw your attention back to the breath.

7. Now place one hand on your belly and one hand on your chest. Bring your awareness to your chest. Do you feel your breath expanding both your chest and upper back as you breathe in? Do your ribs also flare out to the sides? Are there any areas where your breath is unable to move freely?

8. Bring your awareness to your belly. As you breathe in, do you feel the front of your belly lifting? Do you feel the breath causing movement in your lower back? What about your pelvic floor: can you feel it moving with your breath?

9. Are there any other descriptions of your breath that come to mind? Feel free to be creative.

10. Take a few minutes to continue your exploration, then slowly and gently roll to one side and come back up to a seated position.

(Almost all breathing techniques in yoga are done through the nose. If you are stuffed up, you can do this exercise with your mouth slightly open.)

A Note from Katrina

If you practice this exercise every day for two weeks, as I did, following Alan's instructions, you will soon become more aware of your breathing patterns. You will find that they change according to the time of day and your emotional state.

I noticed that, first thing in the morning, when I was relaxed, my breath was smooth and even; but later in the day, if I was feeling stressed, it became shallow and choppy. You might experience something similar.

The exercise can be done whenever you like: try experimenting with it at different times. By studying the breath, you will learn to identify when your breathing is not working to your best advantage. This self-study (*svadyaya* in Sanskrit) is the essence of the yogic practice; through *svadyaya* you can begin to identify the patterns and tendencies that are keeping you bound up inside, and find the freedom that is yoga.

After only a few days of practice, I was sleeping better. And then a funny thing happened: on one of my fat days, I had another craving for pizza, but this time I actually went ahead and ordered it instead of forcing myself to have salad. I ate it, enjoyed it, and then waited for the guilt and shame to overwhelm me. Nothing! I felt great! Absolutely a first for me.

As you practice with the breath, you will experience changes particular to you: they might be subtle at first, and you may not notice them immediately, but the more you practice, the more control you will gain over your breathing—and eventually over your life.

The breath is a powerful tool. If you have not worked with it before, be prepared to experience some unusual side effects: as the breath moves inside you for the first few times, you may become emotional. Or you may simply fall asleep.

Your body is responding. Big changes are coming.

The journey is just beginning.

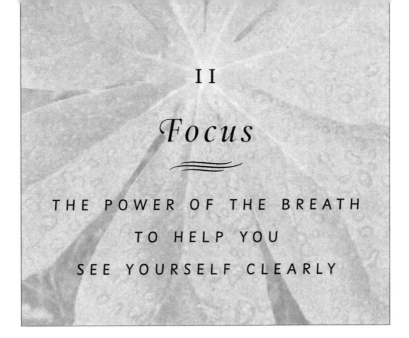

I I

Focus

THE POWER OF THE BREATH
TO HELP YOU
SEE YOURSELF CLEARLY

"What's wrong?" Matthew said. After living with me for five months, he knew when I was "playing up," as he called it.

I continued to stomp around the room, muttering. Couldn't he see that I was in the early stages of an acute anxiety attack?

"Oh, the usual stuff." I tried to sound light. "How hard it is for me to be dependent on you financially. And wondering when you are going to tell me that things are over between us." I'd be alone. Utterly alone. In the big city. What would I do then?

"You don't understand how vulnerable I feel," I added for effect.

I was holding a DVD of *The Big Sleep*. Matthew was writing an essay on it. On the cover, Bogart and Bacall stared at each other. On closer inspection, I could see that they were staring past each other. And when I looked really closely, I could see that they weren't even embracing—they were trying to throttle each other!

Matthew took the case from me and popped the DVD out. "Well, schweetheart," he said, doing his best Bogie, "I have no plans to get rid of you . . . yet."

"Not funny." Didn't he take anything I said seriously?

Matthew sighed. "We've discussed this a million times." He put the DVD in the player. "If you prefer to go back to Calgary and get a full-time job in marketing, then I'll understand, but I think you should give yourself—and me—a chance."

He turned on the player. If there was one thing about Matthew that infuriated me, it was that he would end a conversation just as I was getting started.

"You're not helping," I said. "And it's really bothering me that you don't care to discuss it."

"But I do!" he said.

"Then *talk* to me."

"But I *can't* when you're like this." Now there was more than a hint of impatience. "You close off, and nothing I say makes any difference. Maybe you should go and practice some of those breathing exercises, and then we can try to have this conversation again."

Okay, that was it. There was only one thing to do now: scrunch up my face and let a few tears fall. Let's see how he handled *that*.

He handled that by turning his attention to the film credits.

I stormed into the bedroom and flopped on the bed. *How dare he say that I'm closed off? I'm totally open. Didn't I uproot my life to move here to be with him? With no security? How many people would have taken such a risk? And what kind of commitment has he made to our future? He hasn't proposed once!*

None of this made me feel any better. I could hear the movie starting. Should I go back in? I had been looking forward to watching it. But I couldn't. That would be an admission of defeat. It would send a clear message that I was in the wrong. And I wasn't!

So I buried my head in the pillows and tried to squeeze out a few more tears, and when that wasn't happening I rolled over onto my back and stared at the ceiling.

> Q: Why do I have to argue with Matthew when he is so supportive?
> A: Because he hasn't asked me to marry him.
> Q: But do I really want to get married?
> A: I don't know. I never wanted to before.

Thoughts of marriage turned to thoughts of my mother. How she had been given an "allowance" each week by my father. And how, when she was fifty-two, her marriage had ended and she had been forced to get a job and struggle to make ends meet after staying at home for fifteen years to look after her kids. Having witnessed her go through that, why on earth would I want to get *married*?

I forgot all about breathing. I closed my eyes and gave myself up to a full-scale panic attack. This whole situation just wasn't working.

———

In the days immediately after my first class with Alan, I had practiced hard. I wanted him to think I was a good student.

I could hardly wait to do the exercise for two weeks and then run back to him with a report on how much progress I had made and how my life had dramatically improved.

And at first I did feel different: definitely more relaxed and certainly more confident. For the first time since I moved to New York, I felt that I was doing something worthwhile. My life was progressing in a positive way, which was exactly what I wanted.

But then, after a week had gone by, I hit a roadblock. Instead of the exercise becoming easier, to my astonishment it became *harder*. I soon became angry when I could not feel the breath flowing through me the way I knew it was meant to. So I stopped. I hate to admit it, but it was just like me to give up on something new when it required extra effort. Before long my head filled up with more and more negative thoughts. I was right back where I started.

Which was probably why I couldn't stop arguing with Matthew.

I wished I could talk to Alan, but I just didn't know him well enough yet. And I couldn't call home to pour out my complaints because that would give everyone the satisfaction of knowing I had made a huge mistake.

I was on my own here.

"Come on, you," I told myself, "for just this once don't give up at the first fence and run in the opposite direction. Stay with it."

———

So in the week after our blowup, I tried to be extra nice to Matthew to show him how much I appreciated everything that he was doing for me. The air began to clear. I started to feel better about things.

Then one day I came home to find him as usual tapping away at his laptop. He was working on an essay, I assumed. But I also noticed that he was flicking back and forth from the document to a financial markets website. In one of our many conversations about money, he told me that he had lost quite a lot in the stock market. On a list of things I least wanted to hear, this was pretty close to the top. Now I was worried that he wouldn't have enough to pay for his master's degree. Or next month's rent. Or to support me.

And there he was, doing it again. Flick, flick, flick. The old knot in my stomach, which had untied itself for a couple of days, twisted itself tighter. I had to say something. But then we would have another argument, and I didn't want that. I just wasn't strong enough at the moment.

Straightaway my thoughts drifted back to home. Maybe I should have stayed with David after all. I pictured myself decked out in the latest Juicy Couture on the doorstep of our luxury four-bed home, blowing a kiss to him as he left for work in his Jeep Cherokee. After a leisurely morning devoted to bettering myself in some small way (a long bubble bath, for example), followed by a yoga class, I would change into something new and then drive downtown in my black BMW for a lunch date with one of my girlfriends. I'd subscribe to *Wallpaper* and have back issues of *Elle Decor* fanned out symmetrically on the coffee table in the living room.

Glossy images of designer marble-and-granite bathrooms, built-in turbo washers and dryers, and heated three-car garages filled my head. Vases of freshly cut flowers graced every table. That was what I really wanted—comfort and convenience!

I was horrified, not to say annoyed, at how everything I had been running from had suddenly turned back into my fantasy lifestyle. At least I knew enough not to start an argument with Matthew right then. Scowling at our cramped one-bedroom apartment, I grabbed my yoga mat and left, shutting the door just a little too hard behind me.

Even though I'd stopped doing the breathing exercises and hadn't gotten up the nerve to talk to Alan about my "progress," I had dropped by the studio a few times and taken classes with a couple of the other teachers. I had also begun to socialize casually with some of the people I had met in class. There was one girl I was particularly interested in getting to know better: Romilly was a tall, gorgeous blonde who, even when sweating through a series of difficult poses, never lost her chic. She was just the kind of New Yorker that I had hoped to befriend—maybe hoped to become. After a couple of hellos, we had arranged to get together for coffee.

I met Romilly in City Bakery, just off Fifth Avenue. Thanks to my scrupulous study of fashion magazines, I knew right away that the Marc Jacobs bag she was toting was this season's and cost around a thousand dollars. I was embarrassed to be holding something I had bought on sale in Canada. I hid it under the table.

She sat down. People looked. She basked. Then we ordered decaf skinny lattes. She wanted to know about my situation with Matthew. I laid out my worries. She listened, but whenever a new man came through the doors her eyes wandered.

"Do you love this guy?" she asked distractedly at the end of my report.

"Sure. I mean, of course."

"You can do better," she said.

"In what way?"

"Manhattan is full of rich, successful men. You don't need

to hang out with some guy who is losing money. And you *definitely* don't want to be around when he's lost it all. Look, don't worry. I can introduce you to people."

Romilly told me all about her own plans for the future. She was going to leave her position as account executive at an advertising agency as soon as she got married and go to work for a charity—saving the Galápagos was her special interest. What she wanted—no, absolutely had to have—was a trust-fund guy with heart. She made it sound so appealing that I thought maybe I wanted one, too. Then I could live in New York, find myself, and have all the luxury, security, and safety I had ever desired.

We finished our coffees and went our separate ways: Romilly to get some fresh highlights, and I to the yoga studio to take a class. Our conversation, though enjoyable, had left me unsettled. Was finding a man with money really that important to me? No. Or I would have stayed with David. But how much money did one need? And why didn't I have the confidence that I could earn it myself?

I can't quite explain why, despite these questions of financial insecurity whirling around in my head, I felt compelled to enter a smart shop, flip through a rack of designer dresses, and whip out my American Express (strictly for emergencies) card in order to buy the slinky black number that was marked down to a mere $125. Perhaps Romilly's status bag was still fresh in my memory. Or perhaps it was the dressing-room fantasy I had while trying it on, in which one of Romilly's multimillionaire friends was staring at me from across the room at a crowded cocktail party and came over to say that he knew from the moment he saw me I was the woman with whom he wanted to spend his life. In reality, this kind of overture would immediately tell me that he was looking for nothing more than a one-night stand, but for the purpose of this highly pleasurable visualization I was prepared to overlook that.

When I arrived at the studio, I asked Charlie to stow my shopping bag behind the counter while I was in class. Before I could stop her, she had pulled the dress from the bag.

"Veeeery sexy," she said. "Wear it without a bra, I dare you."

I was about to say "not a chance" when I realized, to my dismay, that Alan was standing right behind me.

"Big date?"

"Oh no, Alan, nothing like that. It was on sale. I bought it on a whim. This isn't the kind of thing I usually wear. I mean, I'm not the sort of girl who wears stuff like this."

That I felt the need to explain myself said it all. This dress would be another of those sale purchases that should have stayed in the shop, along with the pair of Prada sandals that were half price and so uncomfortable I couldn't walk two feet in them, and the cashmere sweater set from a shop in SoHo that was still wrapped in its tissue paper and would remain so forever after. Until I could re-gift it.

"Well, if you're not that sort of girl, what sort of girl are you?" Alan asked.

"I don't know," I said. "That's why I came to New York."

"I have some time free right now," Alan said. "Why don't you join me and we can discuss this?"

I glanced at Charlie. She nodded and smiled. All right, then.

Alan's phone began to ring as I followed him into his office. He motioned me to sit and answered the call. Grateful for the chance to collect my thoughts, I sat down on a white wicker chair and studied the room. On one wall was a striking photograph of Niagara Falls. And, nearby, one of a hammock slung between two trees, a beach in the background. Several smaller framed pictures sat on the desk. In a group photo of venerable, bearded gentlemen garbed in loose robes, I recognized a young Alan standing next to an older man.

I sat back and tried to breathe calmly. My mind went blank. Alan's voice hummed in the background.

Suddenly the call was over.

"I apologize for the delay," he said, flipping shut his cell, the latest-generation Motorola, if my eyes didn't deceive me.

I turned to the photograph on his desk, and before I could ask, he said, "Ah, that one was taken at my family home in South Africa. My father is standing on my right."

"And the other gentlemen?" I asked.

"Yogis visiting from India—celebrated swamis. Many came to our home. My father was a well-known yogi. He was my first teacher."

He pointed at the other figures in turn.

"That one is Venkatesananda of the Sivananda lineage, and there is Swami Nishreyasananda, standing behind my father. The gentleman on his left is the famous Tantric Master, Bharati."

I had never heard of any of these gurus, but as soon as I got home I read up about them on the Internet: they were some of the leading yogis of the twentieth century and had been instrumental in introducing yoga to the West. Venkatesananda had been a translator of many important Sanskrit texts. Nisreyasananda had taught everything from yoga philosophy to mantra. And Bharati was a poet who had gone into seclusion for many years and then decided that was not the way to yoga; realizing that we all must evolve together, he came down from the mountains to immerse himself in the study of Tantra and went on to become one of the great teachers.

"You learned from all these gurus?" I asked.

"Yes, they taught both me and my father."

Now I felt really inadequate. Compared to Alan, I was as spiritually evolved as a mollusk.

Alan's voice jolted me out of my thoughts.

"Have you been studying your breathing patterns since our class together?"

"I tried my best."

"Does that mean you've stopped?" Alan said, with half a smile.

"Kind of."

"It's always difficult in the beginning, but you must keep at it. To take control of your life, you must first take control of the breath. The breath affects every part of you—physical, mental, and spiritual."

If it's so powerful, why isn't everybody doing it?

Alan smiled, almost as if he had heard my thought. Then he reached over and touched my arm. "This is not some fad theory I'm promoting, Katrina. The wisdom that I'm teaching has been in existence for thousands of years, but until a century ago the texts were mostly written in Sanskrit and decipherable by no more than a handful of master yogis."

I was reminded of how alienated I had felt when confronted with the Sanskrit chanting in Nepal. I looked again at the photograph on Alan's desk. The gentle yogis with their long beards—did these strange, ancient-looking men really hold the answers to the questions that I faced today? Perhaps not. But maybe I could still learn how to levitate.

Alan then explained that his goal in life had been to bring yoga into the modern world and, by making the ancient teachings accessible, show how it could become a valuable part of any person's life.

"You don't have to devote your whole life to yoga to benefit from what I teach," he said. "Everything you need is already inside you. All I'm doing is helping you to find it."

"I've been trying to work out who I really am," I said. "But it's so hard to see myself clearly."

Alan nodded. "Go on."

My mind was always scattered, I told him. I spent too much time reliving painful memories from my childhood, experiencing them as acutely as if they had all happened yesterday. And I also fantasized about a wonderful future in which I was rich and happy and loved and beautiful. But I could never just see myself as I was right *now*.

"Drifting between the past and the future is a common problem," Alan said. "You're neither here nor there, and therefore it's difficult to locate your true path in life."

He was right. That was *exactly* my problem. I was paralyzed by all the images in my head.

"The breath can help you unite the past and future," Alan continued, "so that you begin to really live your life in the present. I can show you, but first I need to know more about your breathing patterns."

I remembered lying on the floor in the yoga studio and having a hard time breathing into my chest and upper back. When I had tried to force my breathing, I became uncomfortable, even anxious.

Alan nodded when I told him this. "Something is inhibiting the breath, then—a blockage."

He asked me to think of all the times during the day when

I might create tension in my back or chest. I thought of the years I had spent hunched at a desk, staring at the computer. Of all the overstuffed backpacks I had lugged about. And the many hours of slouching in front of the TV.

"What are you saying—that I just need to sit up straight?" I tried to stretch myself taller in the chair. Was the answer really so simple?

"Hunching could be a factor," Alan said, "but I am inclined to think that the tension in your upper back and chest is just as likely to have been caused by something mental rather than physical."

I slumped back down. I should have known it wasn't going to be simply a matter of practicing good posture.

"If you're clinging to emotions and can't let go, then your heart closes off, and this sends tension through your chest. You literally don't have room to breathe," Alan said. "The disabling emotions that bind the heart and stifle proper breathing often stem from past grief. Do you still grieve for something, Katrina?"

Grieve? I certainly had a well-worn list of *grievances*: my parents' divorce, my anger at my body, the guy who dumped me in seventh grade, the boss who didn't like the way I stapled. And many others. I started to list them, but Alan stopped me.

"No, I don't want details," he said. "We're not here to resurrect the pain of the past; we're here to open you up inside and free your heart. If we succeed, the past will look after itself. What's important is to release the old emotions, wherever they come from, and allow the process of change to begin."

Alan explained that the more open your heart is, the more accepting you become of the past, and the less you blame others—and yourself. As the capacity of the heart grows, so does your compassion and understanding.

"Once you free yourself from the past, you will begin to see yourself more clearly—and that will solve the problem of the future. You will begin the process of becoming the person you want to be," Alan said.

He glanced at a small silver clock on his desk. "I have only a few more minutes, but there is an exercise that I think will help you a great deal," he said. "May I show it to you?"

———

Alan took a towel and rolled it tightly into a long tube. He placed the towel on the floor and had me lie down so that it was positioned just beneath my shoulder blades.

My head, shoulders, and arms rested on the floor above the towel (with my arms bent at right angles, as if to surrender), my lower back and legs below.

"Now, close your eyes and mouth, and bring your awareness to the breath. Feel what's happening in your body. Pay attention to both the emotional and the physical sensations."

Alan was silent while I continued breathing. Then he said: "Think of yourself as a sculptor and the breath as a chisel with which to chip away at this big block inside you, until we have uncovered the shape of the true you."

I could feel the difference immediately. Having the towel underneath my shoulder blades and my arms above my head made it easier to breathe.

My heart already felt more open, and I said so.

"Excellent," Alan said. "Now I want you to make the breath even fuller. On your next inhalation, please keep your abdominal muscles engaged to prevent your belly from protruding and move the breath more into your chest and upper back."

I followed his instruction—and felt the breath opening my chest even further. I tried to concentrate on moving it into my upper back as well and was amazed to find that it felt as if I was massaging myself from the inside out. My muscles were relaxing more with every new breath.

Suddenly I felt such a wave of sadness rising up inside me that I was sure I was going to cry.

"If you're feeling strong emotion," I heard Alan saying, "try not to get involved with it. Let it go and draw your awareness back to the breath."

For about ten minutes I continued to breathe deeply, and with each breath I could feel myself opening up a little more. I experienced a range of emotions: anger, disappointment, anxiety, self-reproach. Each time I consciously brought my awareness back to the breath and the emotion dissipated.

Then I heard Alan calling my name. I had fallen asleep in the middle of a life-changing exercise. How embarrassing.

"Don't worry," Alan reassured me, "it's quite normal when you start changing the course of the breath. Experiencing strong emotions while opening up parts of you that have been closed off for many years can be exhausting."

Alan told me to roll over onto my side and then, when I was ready, to remove the towel and roll onto my back again.

With the release of emotion, a feeling of warmth and contentment flowed through me. I thought of Matthew, and how fortunate I was to have him in my life. I felt so much more open and free. And grateful for all that I had. But already I was thinking: *How long will this feeling last?*

Alan stood up. "That is all for today," he said. "Practice the technique as much as you can. The more you do it, the more open your heart will become. Don't give up, Katrina. Let the breath begin to reveal the true you."

I left with a new resolve to persevere with the lessons.

If I had wanted proof that Alan had a special power, I had it now. I could feel it in my heart. For the first time in my life, I made a silent vow to stay with something until I had learned everything there was to know. This was my chance to change. Perhaps the only one I would ever get.

I wasn't going to blow it.

Breath Focus 2:
UNLOCKING THE HEART

Time: 10–15 minutes

Props: tightly rolled blanket or towel

1. Place a tightly rolled blanket or towel on the floor. Lie down on your back with the towel or blanket just underneath your shoulder blades. Your head and shoulders should rest comfortably above the towel, your lower back and legs below. If you experience any discomfort, make the roll smaller.

2. Place your arms on the floor (bent up at right angles) on either side of your head. Close your eyes.

3. Breathing through your nose, take a few minutes to notice how your breath is moving in your body and whether any emotional or physical sensations arise. If they do, try to be present with the experience, without judging it in any way.

4. At the end of your next exhalation, engage your abdominal muscles to draw your belly toward your spine. Continue to hold in your belly as you inhale (it may expand a bit), and when you exhale, focus on drawing it in again. Keeping the belly engaged as you breathe will move the breath into your chest and upper back, elevating your rib cage. Try to direct the breath to areas that are especially tight and rigid, gently sculpting your body and creating space from the inside.

5. Stay in this position for five minutes, remaining focused on the breath. Then roll to the right side and take the towel or blanket out from beneath you. Lie back down and notice any changes in your body. Does your chest feel more open? Does your heart? What are you experiencing right here, right now?

A Note from Katrina

Following Alan's instructions, I set a rolled towel over my yoga mat, but at first the towel was too thick, and I had placed it too far down—I felt discomfort in my lower back. I readjusted it, but then it was too high up, and my head and shoulders couldn't rest easily on the floor. After several attempts I found the right spot, and after that I knew the exact position needed for my body.

It is important to make sure that the towel is the right thickness (which will vary, depending on your size and how open you are), and that it is placed directly beneath your shoulder blades. You will know if it is correctly positioned, because you will be comfortable and your chest will immediately feel more open and free. If there is any discomfort in your neck, place a cushion under your head.

Alan advised me to do this exercise for a full month, because of my very tight chest and upper back, and the overflow of emotion I was experiencing.

Now that I have learned to unlock my heart, I am capable of expressing more love, understanding, and compassion for myself and others. And I have let go of many of the old, painful feelings that were gnawing at me.

Of course, there are still times when I think of the past and dream of the future. It would be impossible not to. But, thanks to this exercise, my thoughts no longer have the power they once did to confuse and distract me. I can see myself more clearly.

I have learned to live in the *now*.

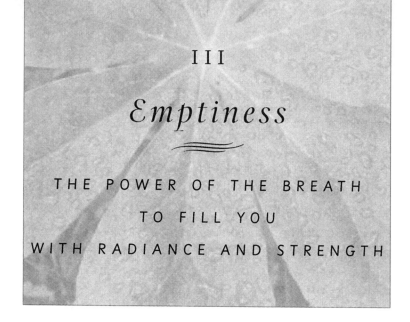

III

Emptiness

THE POWER OF THE BREATH
TO FILL YOU
WITH RADIANCE AND STRENGTH

It was a Wednesday morning and I was on my way to visit Alan. He'd just moved to a new apartment, and since I had time on my hands, I'd offered to help him unpack and organize. Maybe I wasn't yet able to put my own house in order, but I knew I could do a good job of it for someone else.

On my walk over, it crossed my mind that this was New York, and maybe I shouldn't just accept the invitation of someone I didn't know that well. But I felt comfortable with Alan and had good reason for wanting to lend a hand: I was eager to give my progress report on the last breath exercise he had shown me. I'd been faithfully "unlocking the heart" for fifteen minutes every day. And I really thought I could feel something changing inside. It was exciting. But slow. I was doing my best not to be impatient, but I wished the new me would hurry up and make her appearance.

While doing my breathing, taking yoga classes, teaching at FIT, or arguing with Matthew, I continued to ask myself the questions *Who am I? What is my purpose?* And I still couldn't come up with answers. Meanwhile, the days just seemed to shrivel up and blow away, like the old scraps of paper that littered the sidewalk. I shivered and pulled my scarf more tightly around my neck. How could anyone find enlightenment in this dreary environment, anyway? If it were up to me, I'd abolish February and move straight to March.

I arrived at Alan's apartment and rang the buzzer. His new place was in the heart of the East Village, an area that used to be a magnet for artists and young people because it was so cheap. And at one time it had been notorious for drugs. In nearby Tompkins Square Park, so my guidebook claimed, the first outdoor chanting of the Hare Krishna movement had taken place, back in 1966. Knowing all this, I had somehow expected to find Alan living in an old walk-up apartment or bohemian loft with a pull-down fire escape. But his apartment was part of a modern condo complex whose dusty pink walls had a whiff of Miami about them. And there was a brand-new, highly rated restaurant on the corner. Not a Hare Krishna in sight.

Before we began unpacking, Alan made me a pot of fresh tea—real English tea, which he bought from a little shop in the West Village—and told me to sit down on his large, comfortable, fabric-covered sofa. I slowly sank into it, grateful for the mushy softness. I could have fallen asleep right there and then; it had been one of those nights when my overactive imagination had teamed up with my irrational fears to produce a horror movie for my personal entertainment. Last night's was called *99 Ridiculous Ways to Die*:

* While on the toilet, I am bitten in half by a crocodile that has found its way out of the sewage system . . .
* While standing at the foot of the Empire State Building, I am brained by a penny thrown from the observation platform . . .
* While poking my head out of an express train window, I am decapitated by a train coming the other way . . .

All totally *ridiculous*. But what could I do? Once my mind started racing, it wasn't a sprint, it was a marathon.

Alan's living room, which also contained his office space and a built-in kitchen, backed onto the building's courtyard. There were half-opened boxes right and left, and stacks of books piled high: art history, Eastern philosophy, landscape and portrait photography. Carved wooden deities, tribal masks, and several smooth stone figurines were sitting on the coffee table. Although by New York standards the room was spacious, back in Calgary it would have been used as a storage container.

"I didn't know you were a collector, Alan," I said, gesturing to the objects on the coffee table.

"I'm not, really. But sometimes I see something, and it speaks to me. That mask over there, for instance—"

"Spoke to you?" I asked.

"It said, Buy me."

"Very funny, Alan." Ha ha huh.

"Seriously, though," he said, "tribal masks, stone statues—they are the repositories of their people's fears and prayers. Think of all that bottled-up emotion they hold inside."

I inadvertently let out a big sigh.

"I see you have some bottled-up emotion of your own," Alan said. He studied me. "Your aura is very faint. Indeed, it is scarcely visible."

I smiled at him. *You're kidding, right?* The look on his face said he wasn't. I scanned the objects on the table, racking my brain for a way to make light of my gaffe. I gave up and met his gaze once more. He was looking at me thoughtfully now, maybe even with concern.

"Katrina, your aura tells me everything. I can see that you feel listless, lackluster—"

"Oh?"

"—and rather lost."

I silently cursed the aura I didn't believe in for betraying the sad truth about me.

"Have you been doing your breathing exercises?"

"Of course I have! And I'm making progress, I think—but how can I be sure? If the exercises really work, then why do I feel so, I don't know, *empty?*"

I wasn't sure if that was the right word, but it was the only way I could describe how I felt. I wished now I had said nothing. This was definitely not the conversation I had imagined. My plan had been to impress Alan with my diligence and commitment—to demonstrate that I was worthy of his time and attention.

But Alan didn't seem disappointed with me. "Do you often feel like this?" he asked.

I admitted that I did.

"And what happens then?"

With anyone else I would have glossed over my feelings, but I felt compelled to tell Alan the unvarnished truth. I admitted to having dark moods, and confessed that even though I knew I should be thankful for everything I had, it never seemed to be enough. Then, with a combination of shame and defiance (my specialty), I revealed one of my most awful secrets: "When I'm depressed, I eat. Last night, if you can believe it—I know Matthew didn't—I polished off almost a pint of Ben & Jerry's Cherry Garcia."

I braced myself for a scolding. *You need to control yourself. To be grateful for your blessings. To do better.* After all, wasn't Alan a Master Yogi? Wasn't yoga about personal discipline?

To my astonishment, Alan just smiled sympathetically. "That Ben & Jerry's is a killer," he said. "But food can never fill up the kind of emptiness you are talking about."

He was so right. Food used to work, though. Or clothes. Buying something new to wear always made me feel better. For a while. And I'd sat through thousands of hours of bad movies and pointless TV shows, trying to fill the void. But the old tricks didn't seem to cut it anymore. And there were moments when I felt worse than ever.

I related all this to Alan.

"Buying something new to wear, going to the cinema— they are hardly crimes, Katrina, merely distractions. But as you see," Alan continued, "the real problem remains unsolved."

I wondered what the real problem was, and if it could ever be solved. What if I was incapable of true happiness? What if *I* was the problem?

"Why do you think I feel empty?" I said, hoping that my feeble aura had nothing to do with it.

"Because you are searching for something," he replied. "And, in a way, that is good: it means you are looking for change. The problem is that when your mind casts about for—but cannot find—what it needs, it tries to settle for what worked in the past, and tells you to eat or shop. But those things are no longer effective."

In a flash I realized the truth: I wanted to change, but my spirit was only too eager to settle for the instant comforts that had appeased it in the past.

"I don't know if I can overcome my weaknesses," I said.

"This has nothing to do with weakness, Katrina. That word is used far too often, and it has done a lot of damage. If you do not know what you need to be fulfilled, how can you blame yourself for not finding it? Right now, it is enough that you feel this emptiness, and that you want to do something about it. This feeling is not a curse or a failing—it is a blessing! It signals *change*. You have begun your journey to fulfillment. Now is the moment to accept that you cannot pacify yourself with possessions. Not that there is anything wrong with having things, as long as you don't let them have you! But you need to find a more lasting contentment."

Did he think I hadn't already tried? I told him about the years of therapy I'd undertaken and the boxes of self-help books I'd read. I even admitted that I'd tried hypnosis.

"And did it work?" Alan asked.

"Perhaps at night I run naked through the streets, clucking like a chicken," I said, with half a smile, "but I doubt it. After all my efforts to change, I'm still the same person."

"That's because you have been looking for answers in the wrong places," Alan said. "On the outside instead of in."

"But you said it yourself. I'm empty. I don't *have* anything inside!"

"*Everything* you need is inside, Katrina. And to fill the emptiness you must go inward and make contact with the Divine."

The Divine.

And suddenly I was a child again, kneeling side by side with my granny to pray before bed. Together we would chant: "Now I lay me down to sleep, I pray the Lord my soul to keep. If I should die before I wake, I pray the Lord my soul to take." That prayer had terrified me. Supposing I died in the night and God had not heard me—was I condemned to roast in Hell? Eternally? As a child I had once burned my hand on the hot plate and had never forgotten it. What would it feel like if my whole body was covered in flames?

That prayer, along with the occasional Easter or Christmas service at the local Presbyterian church, was all I had known of religion as a child. Fear and boredom.

Alan saw the look on my face.

"Don't fret," he said, "I am not going to lecture you about God."

Then he told me to forget good and evil, strength and weakness, Heaven and Hell, because these oppositions can create terrible stress in a person. He asked me, instead of seeing God as something outside of myself, to recognize the God *inside*. God was not, he said, some white light, or a gentleman with a long beard, or any of the countless ideas that had been created over the millennia to give form to the Divine.

"God is you. And me. He—or she—is all of us," Alan said. "We are all drops in the great ocean of consciousness that created the Universe."

Oh no, we're back in Crazyland. But this time I didn't smile. This time I'd listen without prejudice to what he had to say. What did I have to lose?

"Think of it like this," Alan said. "An ocean is composed of many drops of water, and those drops are also the ocean. One drop contains the essence of the whole. *We are all part of the Divine.*"

This didn't sound like any kind of religion I'd ever heard of, and I told him so.

"I'm not talking about religion," Alan said, "I'm talking about enlightenment. Not worship, science. The science of Tantra."

Tantra? Wasn't that some kind of toga-wearing cult in which dirty old men initiated young girls?

"Isn't Tantra all about sex?" I said.

Alan laughed. "That's what the media would like you to think."

He went on to explain that the word *Tantra* is a contraction of the Sanskrit words *tanoti* (expansion) and *trayati* (liberation). Unlike many religions, in Tantra the physical world is not seen as lower than the world of the spirit—on the contrary, it is through the body that one can begin to experience the Divine, which exists in all things in this world, as well as beyond it. This idea is reflected in a profound Sanskrit phrase that dates back to the Upanishadic period (c. 600 B.C.): *tat tvam asi,* which means "I am that, that I am," or "I am the Universe, the Universe is me."

"The popular image of Tantra is a distortion," Alan said. "Tantric philosophy says that everything we experience—everything we are—is divine. The science of Tantric yoga gives us the tools to help us recognize this in ourselves, so that each and every moment can be full of joy and possibility."

We sat in silence for a while. This was a lot to absorb, and my thoughts soon meandered to matters less spiritual, such as whether the Korean nail salon I had spotted down the street would have an opening for a pedicure after I finished helping Alan. He seemed to sense that I had lost the thread and suggested that, if I wanted, we could meet again at a later date to continue our talk. I was grateful for the offer; I knew that the more I pondered our discussion, the more questions I would have. I set about helping him to unpack.

Two hours later I sat in the salon with my toenail polish drying, replaying our conversation in my head. Clearly, Alan was a great teacher, and I could learn a lot from him. But was it, well, *healthy* to have a mentor at my age?

Confession time: I have been looking for mentors all my life. The problem began with the respect (perhaps fear is a better word) I have for my father. So much of my childhood was spent trying to please him, but he was not easily pleased—not with me, not with my mother, not with himself, not with life. Unable to win his approval, I have sought it elsewhere, from other, older males: boyfriends, teachers, bosses.

The therapist I was sent to at age sixteen became a surrogate parent; I could speak to him as I never could at home, and he listened and was compassionate. But that could not continue forever.

Then there was a teacher at university, Dr. Corcoran, whom I revered. He seemed to know everything, and I longed to receive his wisdom, so I worked hard and got decent grades. I wanted him to notice me—to give me his blessing. It never happened. At the end of the semester, he put his books and papers into his scuffed leather briefcase, snapped it shut, said goodbye to the class, and left the room.

I followed him into the fluorescent-lit corridor and tried to engage him; all I wanted to do was say how much I had enjoyed his teaching, and how much I would miss it in the future. I can still vividly recall my disappointment as I watched his brow furrow while he rummaged in his head for my name. I knew he couldn't possibly remember every one of his hundred or more students, but it was terribly important that he remember me. He didn't. Yet again I had failed to make an impression.

I won't deny that I have tried hard to overcome this rather childish tendency to want a surrogate father in my life, and, for the most part, I have pretty much succeeded. But now I worried that Alan had resurrected my dormant desire for a hero. Even while I had practiced my first breathing exercise, I'd secretly imagined him as my guru, solving all my problems and leading me toward complete self-understanding.

———

Life continued as usual for a few more weeks, while I thought about whether or not I should put my faith in Alan. The decision felt momentous to me. I decided to attend one of his regular Thursday classes to see if I could come to a conclusion. During the meditation I found it hard to sit still, but instead of getting up and leaving, I persisted. I was glad I did, because after class I ran into Alan in the hallway.

"Katrina! How are you? I've been thinking about you. Are you as good at taking notes, filing, that kind of thing, as you are at unpacking boxes?"

I had been prepared for all sorts of questions, but not this one. Caught off guard, I simply nodded.

"Good. I've just got to send a quick email and then we'll talk," he said. He went into his office.

"Oh, wow, I think he's going to offer you a job," Charlie said from behind the front desk. "His previous assistant just left for California. She couldn't handle the negativity of the city any longer."

"But he doesn't know the first thing about me!" I said.

"Alan is very intuitive," she replied. "He doesn't need to see a résumé."

A few minutes later Alan opened his office door and gestured for me to come in. I had already decided not to tell him about my little mentor problem. I sat down and prepared to accept his job offer without seeming overeager, but instead he said, "Have you thought more about our conversation on emptiness?"

"Yes, I have," I said, feeling a bit deflated that he wasn't going to employ me after all.

"And you're ready to find the Divine inside."

"I guess so."

"You don't sound very enthusiastic," Alan said.

Should I talk about my "mentor problem" now? Yes. I had to say something. Alan listened as I told him my story, and at the end of the speech he said, "Ah, but I do not see myself as a mentor, so you need not worry."

"No?"

"Whatever you learn from me really comes from inside you. I am only teaching you how to tap into your own power," he said.

At that moment I knew that what Alan could offer me was different from anything I had ever known. He didn't want to control me—he wanted to empower me. What he had to teach me was just what I needed. I told him I was ready to learn.

Alan explained that in the Tantric tradition the navel is considered to be a sacred center of energy. As much as the legs and feet, the belly is an integral part of a body's strong foundation.

"So in order to fill the emptiness," Alan said, "you will breathe into your core, the area around your navel, which will remove restless longings and renew your dedication to life and to yourself."

Doing this would strengthen my stability and reconnect me to the energy, wisdom, and grace of the Universe—the Divine. My feelings of futility, helplessness, and emptiness would simply disappear.

And so my lesson began.

———

Alan asked me to relax and close my eyes, concentrating only on my breathing, which would remove any distractedness and bring me into the moment.

"I want you to focus on making space for the breath to travel down to your navel as you breathe in through your nose," he said. "Then feel the inhalation filling your torso right to the top of your chest. As you breathe out, feel the breath moving back to the point behind your navel."

I began to breathe in and out, concentrating on the ebb and flow.

After a while I could feel my torso opening up, although when I tried to force my breath down toward my belly, I experienced the same uncomfortable feeling I had had that first day in class.

"Certain areas feel tight," I said, without opening my eyes. "I can't seem to direct my breath into them."

Alan reassured me that this was normal; the belly is one of the major areas to tighten up under stress. To counteract the tension, he told me to bring my hands together, as if for prayer, and rub them lightly, creating a little friction. Then he asked me to move my hands about an inch apart and feel the radiant energy—called *tejas*—flowing between them. I did what he said—and was astonished when I could feel something like a soft electrical current in the air between my palms.

"What you are feeling is just a fragment of the energetic force that makes up the entire Universe," Alan explained. "Now place your hands anywhere you sense tension. Feel them transferring warmth and energy to the area, relaxing it and softening it."

Amazingly, wherever I placed my hands seemed to yield. I felt myself opening up more and more.

"Be very gentle with yourself," Alan said. "There is no need to force your breath in any way. Notice any emotion that flares up—there is often an emotional release accompanying a physical one."

My breath began to settle into my belly naturally. I ceased trying to control it. My torso felt like a huge balloon that expanded in three dimensions when I inhaled and emptied completely when I exhaled.

Alan continued to guide me. "Feel the powerful energy center in your abdomen growing brighter with each breath, as if your inhalations and exhalations were fanning an internal flame. Let new, living energy and a vital feeling of power fill the space inside, removing the emptiness and the restless longing that went with it. You are now the center of the Universe, and everything you need is there for you."

As I breathed in and out, tears spontaneously rose to my eyes, and I let them fall without reacting. I felt calm. I felt spacious inside. I felt free. I needed nothing else in the world to make me happy. And I was doing it on my own. I was giving myself what I needed.

Time passed without my being aware of it.

And then Charlie knocked on the door, alerting Alan to his next appointment. I heard him thank her, and then he spoke to me: "Katrina, gently open your eyes and bring yourself back to the present."

I felt great. I tried to tell Alan how much I appreciated everything he was doing for me, but he raised a hand. "Well, now you can do something for both of us. My assistant Annemarie has left me, and if there's one thing that Tantra can't help with, it's paperwork. I'm hopeless at it. Come and work with me, Katrina, if you really want to learn more about yoga."

I said yes. Of course. And went home exhilarated. This carried through to the next day, so in the morning I went to The New School to enroll in a course. And waited in a long line to register—without bolting, a sure sign of my commitment. I had contemplated photography or drawing but decided on creative writing. I had wanted to continue my writing after university, but back home it was difficult; I was always too busy, and there wasn't much in the way of evening classes.

What had Alan said to me? The emptiness signaled a desire for change.

I had that desire for change. I'd had it for a long time.

And now, at last, I was doing something about it.

Breath Focus 3: CORE BREATHING

Time: 10 minutes

Props: pillow or bolster for under the knees if your lower back is tender

1. Lie down comfortably on your back. Position pillow or bolster as needed. Close your eyes and mouth, and simply follow your breathing for a minute or two.

2. Focus on your inhalations. As you breathe in through your nose, make space for the breath to travel down to your navel, and then feel the inhalation filling your torso up to the top of your chest (allow your belly and chest to expand), all the way to your collarbones. If you sense that there is any tension inhibiting you from reaching full capacity, rub your hands together very gently, creating heat and friction. Draw them about an inch apart, feel the radiant energy in between (*tejas*), and then place them on whichever part you need to release.

3. Now focus on your exhalations. As you breathe out, feel the breath moving back to the point behind your navel. At the very end of the exhalation, contract your abdominal muscles to bring your belly in toward your spine and draw your pelvic floor up (which for women feels similar to Kegel exercises). Concentrate on your strength and power.

4. Practice twenty to thirty breaths in which the breath moves from a point behind the navel up to the collarbones on the inhalation and back down on the exhalation. Let these full breaths fan your internal fire, filling you up with personal magnetism. To intensify this experience you can place your hands one on top of the other and circle them around your navel (counterclockwise for women, clockwise for men).

5. Notice your entire abdominal area. Focus on any special sensations of warmth, comfort, and energy. Remember them for the future.

6. Allow your breath to return to normal. Roll over onto your right side. Open your eyes, resting in that position for a few moments; and then come back up to a seated position.

A Note from Katrina

Alan suggested that I practice this breath for a few weeks, until I was completely at home with it. I would usually spend ten to fifteen minutes on each session. This exercise greatly increased my breath awareness, as well as removing feelings of emptiness. Using the image of a balloon inflating and deflating inside me helped to maximize the benefits that this breath has to offer.

Whenever I feel an urge to do something on the spur of the moment (that I know I will regret later)—eat something stupendously bad for me, or buy that dress or those shoes I know in my heart I will never wear—I use this breath to take away the feelings of restless longing. Core Breathing is also very relaxing, which makes it an excellent aid to winding down at night; I often use it before bed, when I am feeling hyper. By concentrating on the breath for a few minutes, I have found that even an overactive mind like mine can be quieted long enough for sleep to take hold.

After I had tried for so long to find the answers on the

outside, hopping from one short-term solution to another, what Alan showed me in this lesson came as a great comfort. The search started and stopped with me: I held the key to my own problems. And now I knew how to use it.

Tantra teaches that you do not have to deny yourself the pleasures of living; what Core Breathing can do is show you that you need not be governed by the desire for instant gratification. By making contact with the Divine within, you instantly remind yourself that you are a part of the Universe, and it is a part of you.

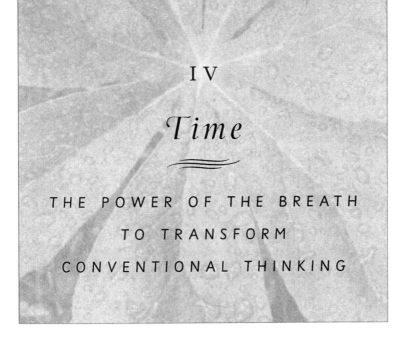

IV

Time

THE POWER OF THE BREATH
TO TRANSFORM
CONVENTIONAL THINKING

"Hey, wanna grab a coffee?"

The morning yoga class had just finished and people were rolling up their mats. I was still supine and in a luxurious free-floating daze when the guy on my right broke the spell. Although I had tried not to notice him during the class, it was impossible to ignore his non-stop grunting and sweating. After months at the studio, I was familiar with the type: the young, overconfident male who treats yoga like a contact sport, always forcing himself deeper into the poses.

"No, actually, I'm—"

"Because I was watching you during the class . . ."

In spite of myself I felt a flush of pride. My daily yoga

practice was paying off, inside and out. It was nice to be admired. Even by a frat boy.

". . . and I hope you don't take this the wrong way—but I'm totally into older women and you look great for your age. You're what—forty?"

———

When I got home—without the coffee, and I wasn't too gentle about saying no—I went straight to the mirror for a close-up inspection. And did what I always do—what I have done for more years than I care to remember: run through every item in the List of Shame.

1. Hair. *Problem:* My real color is a coppery red. In elementary school they called me "Carrot Top"— a simple but effective taunt. At fourteen it traumatized me into home-dyeing my hair black, to my parents' horror (and my delight. At their horror). For more than ten years I have been a fully paid-up blonde.

2. Skin. *Problem:* Freckles, moles, and other sub- and supradermal blemishes. Fearful of the sun, I am susceptible to flaky dryness from a buffeting wind. My natural habitat should be underground.

3. Physique. *Problem:* I am built for endurance, not for lounging. My most striking features are my calves— perhaps *cows* is a better word. There have been periods in the history of fashion when well-developed calves have been considered sexy—Elizabethan England, for example, although that might have been on the men—but with today's high boots and tight-leg jeans, big calves are nothing but a big pain. Unfortunately, every Canadian activity—skiing, skating, hockey, climbing, hiking—

is conducive to calf enlarging. Growing up, I did them all. I love sports. I hate sports.

I stared at myself some more. The proof was there, right in front of my eyes. Right below my eyes, in fact.

I had wrinkles. *Wrinkles*. At thirty!

I was about to have a good old-fashioned building-to-a-crescendo wail when the phone began to ring. Grateful for any distraction, I turned away from the mirror and flopped down on the bed. I lifted the receiver.

There was a crackle on the line, and then the familiar voice.

"Hello, dear, oh, hold on a minute . . . Oops, can you hear me? Almost lost the—" For a moment I thought the line had gone dead. But no. "There, that's better."

"Mom?"

"Katrina? Is that you?"

I sighed. "Yes, Mom. It's me."

"Did I wake you? What time is it?"

"Wake me? Mom, it's nearly midday."

"Well, *I* don't know how people live in the big city, do I?"

"I didn't mean—"

"You can be very hurtful sometimes, you know."

"I'm sorry."

"Yes, well. How are you? What are you doing?"

"Now? Oh, I was just, um, thinking."

"Thinking? Who has time for that? I've been up since five. That's five, my time."

"Doing what, Mom?"

"Eh?"

"You've been up since five, you said."

"Oh, reorganizing the basement. Getting rid of clutter."

My "mother radar" began to tingle. I had left some boxes at her house, pictures and personal things, rather than bring them to New York with me.

"Not my clutter, I hope, Mom!"

"No, I already told you those boxes weren't a problem. I just need to move some stuff around—it's all getting on top of me. I'm taking some boxes out of the basement and moving them to the garage and taking some boxes out of the garage and moving them to the basement. Douglas is coming over to help, I couldn't do it without him—I've pulled something in my back. No matter. This time I'm determined to get everything organized. How are things?"

"Fine," I said.

"Hmm. I came across one of your old teddy bears and a baby blanket this morning. I thought I might keep them for you for when you have a child."

"Oh, okay. That might not happen for a while."

"Well, don't leave it too long. Women are a lot less fertile after thirty-five. Of course, you shouldn't believe everything you read, even if it is in *Time*. After all, I had your sister when I was forty. And look how well she turned out!"

My sister is quite exceptional, and my mother is very proud of her. So is my father. It's about the only thing they can still agree on.

"Any other news?" I said.

Silence.

"Mom?" I knew there was more. But first, a long sigh from her. I knew that sigh. Oh, how I knew it. I sigh in exactly the same way, try as I might not to.

"I spoke to Diane the other day." Diane was my mother's friend. She was also David's mother. "I hate to tell you this, but better you find out from me than from someone less sympathetic. Are you sitting down? David is getting married."

My heart jumped. At the same time as my stomach lurched. Not a pleasant combination. Imagine the inside of a washing machine during its final spin.

"That was quick," I said, trying not to sound off balance.

"Bit of a surprise, eh?"

"When," I said, closing my eyes, "is the wedding?"

"The summer. A summer wedding by the river, so Diane told me, with a speech by the mayor—he's a good friend, you know—and then off to Italy for the honeymoon. Sounds lovely!"

Italy. I had always wanted to live there, in a Tuscan farmhouse. I could see it now, surrounded by rolling hills, bathed in the rays of a golden sun. The lace curtains, the hens in the yard, a big strong tanned Italian farmhand with thick hairy forearms—

"Hello? Katrina?"

"Still here."

"You're invited, you know. If you want to come. It's understandable if you don't. I know it would be hard for *me* to handle seeing an old flame marry another woman, especially so soon after we had parted. But you can't keep men waiting, can you?"

"Hmm? Look, Mom, can I call you later? I have to go."

"Well, I'll be out from eleven to one with Mary-Louise, we're going for a walk on Lack-a-Berry Heath. And then I'll probably grab a sandwich (something simple like thinly sliced oak-smoked ham on rye with Emmental and salad fixings), and then around two I'll be at Strobel's doing the grocery shopping (it's ten percent off today, first Tuesday of the month, and I do need to stock up)—but I'll be back by four as I want to do some baking: there's a new recipe for low-fat bran muffins in this month's *Martha Stewart Living* (for Douglas, he's been sluggish), and then I'll be home the rest of the evening. Probably. So I look forward to your call. And please be careful, dear, there's been a report in the *Calgary Herald* about the top ten terrorist targets, and nine of them are in New York."

I hung up. Thinking about David left me limp, damp, and shivery. *Oh, God, what had I done? I could have been the happy bride. I could have—*

I flopped back on the pillow. Here I was in New York, with nothing accomplished. A dark and heavy cloud of fatigue and despair hovered over me. It was all so depressing. There was nothing to look forward to. I decided to do the only sensible thing I could think of. Sleep. Even if it was midday.

But I couldn't. That damn phone.

"Katrina, Romilly. Listen, I'm gathering up a few girlfriends for lunch today at Da Silvano. I want you to come."

"Love to, but I'm not feeling very social. I just got off the phone with my mom. She told me that my old boyfriend—the fallback guy—is getting married."

"Another loser out of your life. Great! All the more reason to celebrate. Slap on some makeup and a pair of killer heels—"

"I can't walk in heels."

"Flats. Flip-flops. Flippers. Whatever."

Hmm. I did have that new pair of Uggs (as seen recently in *Elle*, which was all the excuse I needed). I could pair them with my supersoft, faded Diesels and a sweater. After a quick shower.

"I'll do my best," I said.

"Good. One-thirty. Now wash that man right out of your hair."

When I arrived at the restaurant a short while later—hair still damp, but the man not quite washed out—Romilly and her friends were already lounging at a table near the back of the room. The three of them looked so stylish and gorgeous that I almost turned around and walked out. But my rumbling stomach wouldn't let me.

Romilly waved me over and introduced me to Thea, an editor at one of the big publishing houses, and Saffryn, who was doing her master's in drama at NYU. I had barely settled myself in my chair when Romilly announced to no one in particular: "Katrina just found out that her ex is getting married."

"Regrets?" said Thea. When I'd come over, she had been jotting in a notebook. Would I end up in there, too?

I tried to sound casual. "He would have been perfect if I had wanted to play wifey." I paused for effect. "Now I'm with someone quite the opposite: a writer."

I should have let it go at that, leaving the girls to wonder about my mysterious, artistic lover. But I added, hoping to sound interesting: "Although I'm not sure if that's going to work out, either."

"Why not?" Thea's pen was poised above the notebook.

"Oh, writers . . . ," said Saffryn and rolled her eyes.

I hesitated.

Then Romilly said, "Your secrets are safe with us, Katrina."

What the heck, it would do me good to get it off my chest. I had no one else to talk to, after all. I started off by telling them all about Matthew's infuriating ability to keep his distance in the relationship. I confessed to the girls that I wanted more than just a live-in love affair, even if I couldn't exactly define what that "more" included. I'd left David because he wanted to marry me, settle down, and have children. And now I wanted to marry, settle down, and have children. With Matthew. Who didn't seem very keen on marriage—his parents had had a bad one—and from that I had assumed he didn't care for children, either. Although I hadn't actually asked him yet.

But if he was absolutely against it, I would need to find someone else. Wouldn't I? I looked at the girls. Romilly and Thea were both nodding and looking sympathetic. All right, then. I could tell them about the Baby Calculator:

To have a baby at thirty-five, I would need to be pregnant by thirty-four.

To be married by thirty-four, I would have to meet someone new by the time I hit thirty-three (allowing three months for fun, three months for adjusting to his baggage, three months of living together, and three months for him to acquiesce to my ultimatum).

Of course, having broken up with Matthew, I would not want to choose someone on the rebound, so I would have to allow six months, maybe a year, to get over him. Which meant that I would have to split up with Matthew when I was thirty-one—thirty-two at the latest.

From which one thing was perfectly clear: *I had less than a year left to sort things out with Matthew, or I would have to find another man!*

The other girls eagerly jumped into the discussion, and it became a free-for-all. What did we really want from men? Excitement or safety? Passion or prudence? Family or freedom? In the end I learned quite as much about these sophisticated New York females as they did about me.

Saffryn dated musicians, even though, as she said, you couldn't trust them with the washing-up, let alone your love. They came and went as they pleased, like cats. But at least cats didn't borrow your money and not pay it back—and they usually had better personal hygiene. And now the question that plagued her was this: Having dated so many men who turned out to be losers, would she recognize a winner even if he pledged everlasting love? And how much longer could she guarantee that hot guitarists would go for her? If she didn't get this whole musician thing out of her system soon, would she end up an exhausted forty competing with nymphettes half her age?

Thea was drawn to older men. *Hommes d'affaires,* men of business. The world-weary, wary types, who were usually married. And usually bored. They were great distractions, but she had woken up the other day and realized that all those distractions had added up to wasted years of life. And now her biological clock was sounding a very loud, very persistent alarm. And suddenly she didn't want to be approaching forty and childless.

By the time our little group broke up two hours later, we had bonded as firm friends. Nothing creates more unity among modern women than a discussion about the time we have spent—and misspent—romancing the modern man.

———

It was four o'clock when I arrived at the studio to give Alan the notes that I had been writing up for his forthcoming lecture. The paperwork he hated so much had now been handed over to me, and whereas in previous jobs I had found that kind of thing a crashing bore, because I was so fascinated by Alan's knowledge, I spent a lot of time writing up his notes and rewriting his work. I guess in the back of my mind was the thought that one day his teachings ought to be published. I also recorded his weekly lectures and transcribed them, and handled inquiries from people interested in Alan as a speaker; he was in great demand at yoga conferences and other studios outside New York.

As soon as I arrived he beckoned me into his office to show off his new Mac. After I had been thoroughly overwhelmed by his childlike enthusiasm for all the new features on it, he suggested that we go for a walk to take advantage of the warm spring weather.

"Who knows how long it will last?" Alan asked. Exactly the question I had about Matthew.

"Aren't you too busy to go out now?" I glanced at all the papers scattered across his desk. I'd have to tidy those later.

"I'm never too busy," Alan said.

"But what about your next appointment—or do you have a class to teach?"

I had a guilty pang about taking Alan away from his work. How could he be so free with his time when his schedule was jam-packed with classes, private clients, and everything else?

He just smiled and waved me through the door.

When we passed the reception area, he told Charlie that he would be out for half an hour or so.

"Cool," she said. "Enjoy the day. I'll take messages. The pollen count is way up—you might want to wear masks." She produced two gauze masks from under the counter.

Alan laughed. "Thank you, Charlie, we'll survive, I'm sure."

"Are you *sure* you have time for a walk?" I said.

"Ah, Katrina, don't fall into the trap of *false time*." Alan smiled as he motioned for me to enter the elevator. "There is *always* enough time to do what you want to do. Don't let our culture's obsession with deadlines frighten you into thinking otherwise."

"I don't think it's quite that simple, Al. Time *does* pass, false or not. For example, I just learned that my old boyfriend is getting married."

"How do you feel about that?" Alan asked.

We had left the building and were walking up Fifth Avenue.

"I'm not sure. I guess it has started me worrying about the future again. If I don't settle down with someone soon, I'll become a wrinkly old maid and no one will want me."

Alan stopped suddenly—and had to apologize to the person who had been close behind him and now ran into his back. Then he said, "No! Again, that is *false time* you are afraid of, Katrina."

Perhaps. But I wasn't the only one. There were women at the yoga studio—beautiful, smart women, some still in their thirties—who were getting Botoxed every few months to cover up any signs of aging. They worried about the future, just as I did. Perhaps they hadn't found the ideal partner and were beginning to suspect they never would, or else they were in a relationship and were anxious that a less than perfect face and figure might mean the end of it. False time? Hardly! The future we women had to face was very, very real. I didn't dare tell Alan, but someone had recently slipped me the private number of a celebrated dermatologist, along with the code word I would need to get an appointment. And I hadn't thrown it away, either. I was keeping the number as insurance. Just in case.

After all, Alan didn't study the beauty and fashion magazines.

I wanted to say to him: If youth and beauty are so unimportant, why are these magazines so popular? It was easy to dismiss such things—if you were a man. Physical decline didn't seem to worry men as it did women. It didn't worry Alan, anyway, as far as I knew.

We arrived at Madison Square Park and sat down on one of the smart wooden benches that had been recently installed. There was a young couple on the bench opposite, locked in a passionate embrace. I thought how great it would be to be so young again, and with everything still to come. At that moment they took a breather and the girl looked at me. I wondered what she would think. Did Alan and I look like a couple? An older man with his younger girlfriend? That wouldn't be so bad. What if she thought we were the same age! That would be awful.

I almost laughed out loud. Why was I always so obsessed with what other people might think of me? Forget the past. Forget the future. Be in the *now*. If I could do that, I might have a chance at understanding—even honestly accepting—what Alan was trying to teach me.

"Let's talk about time," he said. "It's just an idea, after all. The concept of years, days, and hours was invented to help man manage his life. But something has gone badly wrong. Time has turned into a monster, and now we live in fear of it. But, you see, *time exists only in the mind*. We need a new way to look at it, and then we can begin to change our views of aging and what we may accomplish in our lives."

"Easier said than done."

"Not at all," Alan said, "if you're prepared to keep an open mind. Think like a yogi: instead of fearing time, embrace it. For yogis, time can never run out. It is *never* too late. We believe that connecting to each breath leads you *closer to your truth.* Looked at this way, chronological age becomes irrelevant."

Alan explained that through the breath I could unite with a consciousness *outside* time—beyond the mental traps that man has unthinkingly created and is now caught in. Instead of feeling that if I didn't hurry I would miss out on life, I must imagine instead that I had all the time I needed to do *everything.*

"When you inhale, you take in *prana*—the yogic word for 'life force.' The more life force you can attract, the younger you will be inside, which will change how you see the world, and how people see you. I will teach you to replace your short, shallow breaths with long, spacious breaths. Then," he said, "you will be able to receive the maximum amount of *prana* with each and every inhalation."

I unconsciously took a deep breath. It was so simple, but I felt better immediately. Supposing I could feel like this all the time?

Alan continued: "To distribute *prana* effectively throughout your system, the inhalation must create movement and space in your whole torso. Now that you have explored the breath in your belly and chest, I want you to experience the breath as it passes through them. A full, complete inhalation."

And I began my next lesson, which Alan called the Fountain.

———

He asked me to start by taking a few normal breaths, inhaling and exhaling all the way. In spite of the distractions—the couple on the bench opposite, the hum of the traffic on the far side of the trees—his voice immediately directed my awareness to the breath.

"On your next inhalation I want you to breathe in three even stages," he said, "with a pause after each one, filling yourself from the bottom up, as if you were a fountain preparing to spout."

I nodded.

"Good. Inhale, expanding your lower belly and back. Pause."

I tried not to breathe in too quickly.

"Continue, expanding your middle chest and back. Feel your ribs flaring out. Pause."

At this point I had to be careful not to let the breath run away from me, in order to have enough room inside for the third stage to fill me up to the top.

"Inhale once more, this time expanding your upper chest and back, drawing the breath all the way up to your collarbones. And pause. Visualize *prana* revitalizing every cell, leaving you pure and vital."

Now I felt as if I were bursting—

"Exhale all the way."

My breath came out with a gush.

"Don't push, just let go. And now pause."

But I had lost control. I was gasping for air. I tried to calm myself and find my focus again, but it took me some time.

"I'm sorry," I said.

"No need to try so hard, Katrina. Let the breath flow up through you like water in a fountain. Just let it happen naturally. If the effort is too great, take a few normal breaths before the next cycle."

When I was ready again, I practiced a few rounds.

Inhale one third. Pause.

Inhale two thirds. Pause.

Inhale to the top. Pause.

I continued to picture myself as a fountain filling up. Exhale all the way. Pause.

And now I really started to feel the flow.

After I had finished, I spent a few moments observing my breath. There was no question about it: my inhalation was fuller, longer, and smoother than it had been before.

"Did you feel your body opening and expanding on the inhalation, drawing the life force into you?" Alan said.

"Not at first—"

"But you had it by the end, didn't you! Make no mistake: this is not a simple breath. Regular practice is necessary to master it. Learn to expand the breath and hold it. Contain it. Fill yourself up with *prana*, and I can assure you of this: it will change your idea of time. When you use this breath, you are going beyond earthly definitions and communing with the Infinite, which is *timeless*."

We stood up and walked through the park to the street. Alan held out his hand to hail a cab, but there were none free.

"I'd better get one soon," he said, "or I'll be late for my next appointment."

"Looks like time does have its limitations after all," I said.

Alan laughed. "Especially heading downtown during rush hour."

Soon after, a cab stopped for him. He waved goodbye, and I watched as he disappeared into the traffic streaming south on Broadway.

Breath Focus 4: FOUNTAIN

Time: 10–20 minutes
Props: none

1. In a chair or cross-legged on the floor, sit up straight. Close your eyes.

2. Take a few normal breaths. Inhale and exhale all the way.

3. Now inhale in three even stages, with a pause after each one (inhale, pause; inhale, pause; inhale, pause). From the bottom up, see if you can direct the breath first into your lower belly and back, then your mid-chest and back, and finally all the way up to your collarbones. When you come to the end of the last pause, hold and feel *prana* revitalizing each and every cell—then let all of the air out of you in one smooth exhalation. Pause. And then repeat.

4. Practice this breath ten to fifteen times, taking in more of the life force with every breath.

5. If you feel out of control, take a few normal breaths after each round to readjust. Don't fret if it does not work the first time. You have all the time in the world.

6. If you find this difficult, consider counting the breaths: for example, breathing in for three counts of three, with a pause after each one, and then exhaling for a count of nine. You can then work up to three counts of four, exhaling for a count of twelve.

7. As you become more advanced, cease counting and just feel the breath.

8. When you are finished, take a few minutes to notice the effects of your practice, with your eyes still closed. Enjoy the feeling of energy and vitality.

≈

A Note from Katrina

You will be amazed at how quickly the Fountain rises through you and flushes away fears of passing time. Thanks to this exercise I have been better able to let go of my tendency to think of time as finite—something there is never enough of.

Alan's exercise not only changed my relationship with time but also changed my relationship with myself. I am now back to my natural hair color (without regrets), and I have a new appreciation for my calves, which, even if I can't stuff them into skinny jeans, allow me to enjoy long hikes, something those matchstick-legged girls couldn't handle without being carried most of the way.

What is it about yourself that you feel uncomfortable with? If you use the Fountain, you may well find that it guides you effortlessly back to the natural and true.

This breath can be used whenever you need to feel rejuvenated, and will benefit your breathing even when you are not practicing it, helping you to absorb more *prana* directly from the Universe.

Alan's advice is to *stop fearing time and embrace it*—the reverse of conventional wisdom. Yoga encourages all kinds of contrary thinking. The headstand, for example, is more than a yoga pose: it is an invitation to turn normal thinking upside down. Even the word *guru,* meaning "teacher," is composed of two words that are the opposites of each other: *gu,* meaning "darkness," and *ru,* meaning "light." A guru leads you from darkness into light. Away from tired, used-up thinking toward fresh and helpful ideas.

While I was learning this breathing technique, Alan told me something that I thought was simply revolutionary:

"A successful life," he said, "means living each day as if it were your first."

"I thought you should live each day as if it were your last!"

He shook his head. "To live each day as if it were your last," he explained, "you would be trying to remedy all the mistakes you thought you had made in your life, all the regrets, all the things undone and unsaid. Whereas if you live each day as if it is your *first*, you are freed from all obligations, all guilt, all regret. And that is why the breath is such a potent tool—it clears away all the accumulated confusion of the years and allows us to begin again. And again. And again."

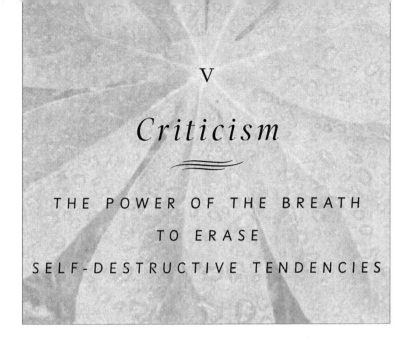

V

Criticism

THE POWER OF THE BREATH
TO ERASE
SELF-DESTRUCTIVE TENDENCIES

"Okay, who's up next? Katrina?"

It was a Thursday evening, and I was at my writing class. Karen, the teacher, was looking at me and smiling. My heart thumped against my ribs.

My turn to read. At last. I'd been working on the story for weeks. I was ready to read it to an audience, wasn't I? That girl Jennie was staring at me. I was breaking into a sweat, I could feel it. I wiped my palms on my jeans, opened my bag, and pulled out my story.

"Okay, everyone, this is a piece called 'The Lantern.' I hope you like it." *I hope you like it.* Why did I have to say that? How dumb. Would my need for approval make anyone like it better?

I reminded myself that this was something I wanted to do. To be a writer, to share my stories. I took a deep breath and started to read.

————

When class was over, my fellow student Lisa, a graphic designer, suggested a drink at Bar Six on Sixth Avenue. Lisa and I had bonded the previous week after I mentioned how much I enjoyed the story about her hippie childhood in Vermont. It turned out that she lived a few streets away from me, just off Greenwich Avenue, and that she was also into yoga. I was glad for the chance to get to know her better.

Bar Six was a passable model of a French café, with a zinc countertop and mirrored wall. It was crowded, as it always was by 9:00 P.M., but we managed to squeeze in at the bar. I ordered a glass of white wine and took a long sip.

"What happened in there tonight?" Lisa asked.

"When Jennie started criticizing my work, I just lost it," I said. "I don't know what came over me." I really couldn't explain.

Perhaps it was a blessing that my inaugural reading was a blur. When I had finished, Jennie, the tattooed and multipierced Amazonian bike messenger (who wrote and read—with great relish—semipornographic pieces about her sex life) slammed into my little story as if she were being paid to destroy it. I went red and almost started to cry. And then I argued back. It was getting quite nasty when Karen finally told Jennie to cool it. That made it even worse: as if Karen felt so sorry for me that she had to intercede on my behalf. I think other people made some comments. I think some of them were even complimentary. I couldn't remember. Only Jennie's scathing criticisms remained in my memory.

"Have you ever had to defend a story like that before?" Lisa said.

"This is the first time I've read my work aloud."

"It's hard to show your writing to other people. It was good," Lisa said. "Really."

"Not according to Jennie—she was very eloquent about its failings."

"Don't let one ignorant person put you off. She's just a kid. Doesn't know what she's saying half the time."

"I'm very sensitive to criticism," I said, hoping we could drop the subject.

"Sensitive to criticism" was an understatement. My sensitivity was like a rose I had grown in secret. A rose with very large thorns.

Lisa bought another round, and then I bought another; I tried to relax and forget about Jennie. Karen had given us a writing exercise to do at home, and I decided I would use it to explore my fear of criticism. Either that or I was going to drop the class. I'd rather quit than risk being pulled apart in front of everyone a second time.

By the time Lisa and I said good night, I'd managed to soothe my aching ego. But the evening's unpleasantness wasn't over yet.

When I got home, I was buzzed from the few glasses of wine and Matthew was grumpy. Not a good combination. Then he said something that really annoyed me, about how I hadn't washed the dinner plates properly and he'd had to do them again. After what had happened in class, I was in no mood to thank him for pointing out any more of my failings. Especially such a trivial one.

"Who cares about the goddamn plates?" I shouted at him. *"Don't treat me like a child."*

Matthew went silent. He was shutting down on me; nothing I could do or say now would salvage this conversation. I had two choices: lick my wounds and retire gracefully, or turn up the heat. All the way up. Until there was a blaze going. We argued for an hour before going to bed exhausted and sleeping as far apart as two people can on a lumpy queen-size mattress. Except that I didn't sleep. Is there anything worse than not sleeping and wanting to make up with the person who is lying next to you and knowing that if you wake him up to say you're sorry he'll scream at you?

———

When Alan called early the next morning and offered to drive me to a meeting at the midtown studio to discuss putting together a new manual for teacher training, I accepted gratefully. I did not want to take the subway, especially after the night I'd had; the crush during rush hour was always uncomfortable—everybody penned in next to one another like cattle going to market—but that morning it would have been unbearable. I was exhausted from clinging all night to my narrow edge of the bed so as not to wake up Matthew, I had a cramp in my neck, and there was a dull, buzzing ache in my head.

I was glad to get out of the house; a few hours apart would be a good thing. I was always ready to make up straightaway, but Matthew seemed to need time to recover from our arguments. We would reconcile when I got home. Or so I hoped.

When Alan's Land Rover pulled up in front of my building, I was standing outside, ready to go. As soon as he stopped, the cars behind his began to sound their horns. In Manhattan you had about five seconds to move before it became an international incident. He opened the passenger side door, and I dashed over and jumped in.

"Good morning!" he said, beaming at me. Car horns didn't bother him. Nothing did. I knew that he had already done his yoga practice before leaving home, just as he did every morning. "Traffic's bad. And I'm hungry. What I wouldn't do for a nice toasted bagel with full-fat cream cheese."

"Well, let's stop then."

He shook his head. "My doctor's put me on a low-fat diet to curb my cholesterol. No more cheese, butter, or chai lattes. For a while, anyway. Until he forgets to ask if I am following his orders."

We stopped at the lights on the southwest corner of Union Square. Alan was looking at me. I tried to arrange my face in a beatific expression to suggest that I, too, had done my yoga practice first thing in the morning and was now enjoying a transcendent inner peace. But at this point Alan knew me well enough to know that something was bothering me. Before he could ask what was wrong, however, I took a deep breath and launched into the expanded, sympathy-inducing version of what had happened in my writing class. It was enough to make the angels weep, I thought, but all he said at the end was "Tell me. Why do you think you reacted so strongly?"

"It hurt, that's why. I put a lot of work into that story, Alan."

"But your reaction seems to indicate something deeper. Almost as if that girl was criticizing you, not what you had written."

"Well, she was," I said.

Alan shook his head. "There's a difference between someone criticizing you and someone criticizing your work, isn't
there?"

*Of course there is, Alan, do you think I'm an idiot? Can't you
see that what Jennie made me feel was not merely that I had written a poor story—but that I would never be a good writer?*

I bit my tongue hard to stop the thought from turning into
speech. What did it take to get Alan on my side? I tried
again:

"But that's not all. When I got home, Matthew was moan-
ing about how I do the dishes. He's always correcting me
about something, and I hate it."

"Oh dear," Alan said.

I turned quickly to look at him. Was that a smile? How
very annoying.

"What? You don't believe me?" I said.

Alan remained silent. He *was* smiling. Or something.
Suddenly, inexplicably, his silence seemed like a challenge.

"Are you saying that this is all *my* fault?" My voice was
rising. "That I'm to *blame?*"

Alan shook his head. "I wish you would not use words
like *fault, guilt, blame,*" he said. "You use them a lot, I've
noticed. I wonder where they come from." He gave me a
sideways look.

"You're not listening to me," I said.

"Oh, but I am," he replied. "And what I am hearing is that
you react very strongly when somebody says something that
you consider to be critical of you. Why, Katrina?"

"Because when someone criticizes me, it reminds me of
my father."

My face was almost on fire. Good Lord, I thought, how
had I allowed myself to get into such a state? I realized with

dismay that my lack of writing and housekeeping skills was not the topic at all.

This was all about my father.

"Tell me about him," Alan said.

So I did. Boy, did I.

I'd never felt good enough for my father. During my teenage years, when I was desperate for his love and approval, I could only remember his angry derision. *I didn't eat correctly. I didn't sit up properly.* And so I gave up trying to please him and instead devoted myself to infuriating him. Because he wouldn't love me for myself, I became someone he would never love. I dressed in ripped jeans and oversize men's coats, and he called me a hobo. I talked with a Valley Girl accent (remember Sarah Jessica Parker in the TV show *Square Pegs?* "Like, gag me with a spoon!")—and he called me a moron. The more he hurt me, the worse I felt—and the more I tried to irritate him. And then I would feel terrible.

But if I told my father how I felt about his criticisms, he would reply that I was too sensitive. Yes, I was. I *still* was. And I had him to thank for it. The irony was that my father was even more critical of himself. But nobody *else* was allowed to criticize him. He was just as sensitive as I was!

I sat back, exhausted. The headache had almost gone. I closed my eyes.

"Thank you for your honesty," Alan said.

I opened them again. "Thank you for listening," I said. "And I'm sorry if I was—"

"Forget it."

That was another marvelous thing about Alan: he never took offense at anything. He actually enjoyed jokes at his own expense; recently he had taken to calling himself the Deluxe Comforter, because he was a bit overweight. Being secure in his own character, he never felt the need to criticize others.

Now we were traveling north up Park Avenue toward the MetLife building. I had another of my death fantasies. In this one, I jumped out of the car into the heavy traffic. A moment of agony and all my troubles would be over. Forever. I fast-forwarded to the funeral. Everyone in Prada black, buckets of black roses, black sunglasses galore (the new Gucci ones). Discreet wailing (dabbing of black lace hankies). Funeral March in B (for black)— flat minor by Chopin. All very tasteful and in grand style.

And then Matthew would stand up to make a speech and ruin everything with a joke about how ironic it was that I got flattened outside one of North America's largest insurance companies when I had absolutely no insurance.

Alan broke the spell. "Katrina," he said, "we are about to enter a rather dark and turbulent area."

"I know," I replied distractedly. "I hate this underpass."

"I am referring to your relationship with your father."

"Oh. Him."

"You have stored up a great deal of his criticism. Over time you have turned that feeling of unworthiness as a child into acute self-criticism in adulthood. This causes you to overreact in certain situations, such as those you faced yesterday in your writing class and at home."

"When I was a child," I said, "I had to do what I was told, but I'm an adult now—I don't have to take any bullshit if I don't want to."

"No, you don't," he said. "But one thing you must understand: the success of your relationships with other people depends more on *you* than on them. The problem is yours."

"*My* problem? But I'm the one being criticized!"

"Are you? Or does all the perceived criticism really come

down to a few unhappy memories of childhood that refuse to go away and are mixed up in your mind with something that happened last week?"

Alan turned off Park Avenue toward Lexington. Then he said, "Whenever you believe that someone is criticizing you, you become a child again—angry, defensive, vulnerable. And powerless. Your only escape, then, is a childish one—you have a tantrum."

I sighed deeply. It was all true. I really felt as if I didn't have a choice about the way I reacted; certain situations automatically triggered these negative responses. It all happened *unconsciously*. Only afterward was I able to retrace events and see how irrational I had been.

We were pulling up in front of the studio. Alan had found a parking space and stopped the car. He always seemed to be able to find a space in this city where people were afraid to move their cars for weeks—years!—in case they lost their spot. He had a special yogic mantra that he repeated to himself: a prayer to Ganesha, the Indian god known as the Remover of Obstacles. Sooner or later, he always found a space. I had witnessed it time and again.

Alan turned off the motor and said, "I know how difficult this is for you, Katrina. But you must be realistic. You cannot control the way other people talk to you. You must learn to distance yourself from an inflammatory situation and understand that the only thing you *can* control is yourself. You are not a child anymore. You are not in anyone's power. Not, that is, until you overreact to something someone says. Don't infuse new situations with old emotions, blurring the issue and turning a trivial matter into a tragedy."

I thought about my confrontations with Jennie and Matthew.

"I don't know how to change," I said. "But I want to."

"That's the first step," Alan replied. "The second step is to use the breath to *create space* in your mind. Then you will be able to distance yourself from the old feelings of conflict, drama, and judgment and see things as they *really* are, free from the distortions of unhappy memories. The need to react violently will disappear."

I tried picturing myself floating serenely through my writing class, smiling graciously as Jennie made one of her barbed comments. *Yeah, right.* But Alan had been right about so many things. I instructed myself to listen without judgment.

"Once you have created space in the mind, the impulse to criticize yourself will, over time, evaporate. You will be able to evaluate what others say dispassionately, without the need to defend yourself or attack the other person. You are conditioned to react in a hostile way, Katrina. We must decondition you."

"That's why I paid for years of therapy," I said. "Which didn't work, obviously. Can I really change this late in the day?"

"All things are possible," Alan said. "The trick is to stack the odds in your favor and make them *probable.* Your self-criticism is too deeply ingrained to be removed by talking with a therapist—although such a course can be beneficial in other ways. But real, physical change can be accomplished by utilizing the breath. In our last exercise we drew in life force on the inhalation; this time we will use the *exhalation* to cleanse your system of impurities."

"You mean expel carbon dioxide?"

"That's part of it. The exhalation does indeed release toxins from the body, but it also helps you to extinguish the negative thought patterns that are toxic to the *mind*. I am going to teach you how to lengthen the exhalation and use it as a tool to release you from your self-destructiveness."

After so many years of feeling trapped by my emotions, I allowed myself to hope. Instead of just talking about the problem, Alan had a practical solution. And if it worked for me, who knew, maybe my dad would try it! He had as much need of it as I did, if not more. And it seemed to be the right time. To my amazement he had recently expressed his own desire to change the things he didn't like about himself.

I listened intently as my next lesson began.

———

"This technique is similar to the Fountain," Alan said, "but this time I want you to reverse the order. Start by taking in a full breath; pause; and then, in three stages from the top down, exhale, pause (let your shoulders, upper chest, and back relax); exhale, pause (feel your rib cage contract); exhale, pause (draw your belly in and pelvic floor up)."

I was so used to practicing the technique on the inhalation that I could do what Alan wanted right away.

"And repeat," he said.

I closed my eyes and practiced a few rounds.

"Visualize the exhalation squeezing toxins and poisons out of you."

Alan told me to keep practicing until my exhalation became long and smooth. Anytime I felt criticism creeping in, he instructed me to expel it with the breath, creating the space inside to distance myself from negativity and purge any lingering painful memories. He said that this breathing technique would help me keep self-criticism at bay until the day when I would find that it had disappeared altogether, leaving no trace of its former occupation.

"This is the next stage toward becoming the person you want to be, Katrina."

I continued to breathe fully and deeply, becoming ever more attuned to the subtle changes in my breath. The sensation was hypnotic, and after a time I noticed that I really wasn't thinking anymore.

My mind was empty, clear.

Because I was really *present*, the past had no hold over me. For the first time in my life I was able to dismiss the old, hostile voices before they could take control.

I had found the space inside.

Without opening my eyes, I heard Alan's voice, as if from far away:

"With every deep, full exhalation, you become more able to *respond* rather than *react*. Your self-criticism is fading away. The more you practice this breath, the less you will need to be the winner and fear being the loser. *There is no right. There is no wrong. There is only being.*"

Suddenly I remembered an experience I had with my father years earlier in India, during the time we were traveling together. Hiking up to a remote mountaintop over Pushkar, we encountered a holy man who told us that I had lived many previous lives as a spiritual teacher and would return to India often during this lifetime, both to learn and to teach. I didn't take it very seriously then, but my dad had subsequently reminded me from time to time of the holy man's prophecy, and that my life might have a hidden meaning. He *did* believe in me. In his heart he loved me and wanted the best for me, as I did for him. We were both victims of our own sensitivity. Or perhaps a better word would be *vulnerability*. But we could do something about it now.

I continued to breathe, feeling all of my anger and resentment—at myself, at Jennie, Matthew, my father, the world—disappearing. I had nothing to prove. I was content. I was free . . .

I was wandering on a wide, grassy plain. The sunshine was warm, but as gentle on my shoulders as the arm of an old friend. I stooped to pick a small yellow flower. The air was fragrant with the smell of pine and fir. Lacy clouds drifted lazily on the horizon. In the far distance, the snowy caps of mountains stood out in a sapphire blue sky. A bird hovered high overhead, resting on the wind currents. There was no one to disturb my peace. I could walk freely for as long as I desired.

When I opened my eyes once more, some five minutes later, Alan was no longer in the car.

He had left the car keys and a note on the dashboard:

Dear Katrina
   Let the breath free your mind and release you from your bondage.
   A

(After our meeting, let's grab chai lattes—don't tell my doctor!)

Breath Focus 5: CASCADE

Time: 10–20 minutes
Props: none

1. In a chair, or cross-legged on the floor, sit up straight. Close your eyes.

2. Take a few normal breaths. Inhale and exhale all the way.

3. Inhale all the way up to your collarbones, letting your belly and chest expand with the breath.

4. Exhale, letting out your breath in *three equal parts* from the top down, pausing after each one: Exhale, pause (relax your shoulders and feel your upper chest and back draw down). Exhale, pause (feel your rib cage contract). Exhale, pause (draw your belly in and your pelvic floor up). Repeat.

5. If you find that you are short of breath, return to normal breathing for a while, and then try again. While you are still learning, it can help to take a normal breath in and out after each round.

6. Continue this for a series of ten to fifteen staggered exhalations, expelling more and more of the self-criticism and criticism of others with every breath. You can visualize a cascading waterfall washing criticism away.

7. Let your breath return to normal.

8. Teach yourself to lengthen the breath by counting. For example: Breathe in for a count of nine, and then exhale in three sets of three equal counts. Or breathe in for a count of twelve, and then breathe out for three sets of four equal counts. Eventually, stop counting and just feel the breath.

9. At the end of the exercise, take a few breaths and notice how the exhalation is longer, smoother, more even.

======

A Note from Katrina

I practice this breath whenever I feel I am being judged. And the more I do it, the less frequently those situations seem to occur. With Alan's help, I am ridding myself at last of those automatic responses to what I think, mistakenly or not, is criticism.

We learn as children that being criticized means we are bad. But we are not bad. It is all conditioning, and we must decondition ourselves. We only need to remember what Alan told me: *There is no right. There is no wrong. There is only being.*

If you feel a crisis approaching, focus on your exhalations in order to release any unhealthy thoughts that are bubbling up. Even doing this for a minute can make a big difference.

I also find this breath helpful whenever I feel myself on the point of overreacting to irritating everyday situations: sitting in a traffic jam, holding for customer service, waiting in line to pay at the supermarket, et cetera. Any time I feel like biting someone's head off for no honest reason. As a result, little problems no longer take up so much of my energy.

You can use this technique anywhere, anytime, even with your eyes open. During any difficult interaction, simply turn your attention to your breath and notice how bad thoughts are instantly dismissed.

There is no one to disturb your peace. You can walk freely for as long as you desire.

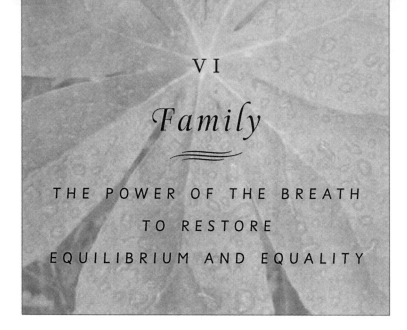

VI

Family

THE POWER OF THE BREATH
TO RESTORE
EQUILIBRIUM AND EQUALITY

"Dad? Dad! *Dad!*"

I stopped waving my arms and watched as the taillights on my father's car faded away into the gloom of Calgary Airport's traffic system. I knew that if I wasn't standing outside Arrivals at the exact moment he drove by, he wouldn't wait. But there was no need to panic; all I had to do was stand in the same spot, and he would come by again in about ten minutes, traffic permitting. Stand in the same spot in freezing weather. Easter in Calgary.

I tried to relax. I watched my breath turn white when I exhaled. *You know there are reasons he hates public parking,* I reminded myself: the long walk from the car, the misplaced parking ticket, getting lost trying to find the way out. Just as there are reasons why he would never be waiting for me outside Customs holding a helium-filled, heart-shaped balloon with my name on it and wearing a look of uncontainable joy on his face. For one, my dad would never buy a helium-filled, heart-shaped balloon, in case one of his buddies from handball happened to be lurking nearby.

Okay, I told myself. *Follow the rules: Stay where you are, whatever happens. Even if your bladder is about to burst. Don't move, don't look away, don't even* twitch. *Be ready to flag him down. You cannot afford to miss him again. He'll be really upset if you do.* (But supposing he had already done a second—or third!—rotation? He'd be ready to explode.)

For some reason the unofficial Calgary Stampede slogan flashed before my eyes. "It's the most fun you can have with your boots on!"

While my left hand slowly froze itself into a claw around the handle of my rolling suitcase, I pulled out my cell phone with the right.

"I'm here," I said, "safe and sound."

"Do I owe you twenty dollars?" Matthew said.

"Yes. He didn't wait."

Matthew chuckled. "Well, what do you know? At least your flight wasn't delayed by the blizzard."

"I'm beginning to wish it had never taken off."

"Do I detect a note of tension?" Matthew asked. "You've been looking forward to going home, try not to upset yourself so soon. You're only there a week, remember."

It was nine months since I'd been back, and I was missing my family. I so wanted this to be a happy homecoming. I was praying that all the work I had done on myself with Alan would pass the test here, where I was most vulnerable to falling back into my old ways. I wanted to be able to re-strain myself when my mother started to talk to me as if I were still the troublesome teenager whose tantrums she had never really forgiven. And if my father was critical, I would try to turn the other cheek. I had to, because I had come to Calgary with every intention of thanking my parents for all they had done for me. I wanted them to see how much I had changed, and then maybe, just maybe, they would change their attitude toward me. And I planned to accomplish all of this in the next seven days.

My father was approaching, flashing his lights. I said a hasty goodbye to Matthew and waved. The car pulled up with a jerk in front of me and Dad got out. The long hug I was hoping for was over in a millisecond.

"Damn traffic gets worse every time I take out the car," he said, picking up my bag and stowing it in the back. In an-swer to my next question, he told me that he had driven by only once. Thank heavens.

The snow was falling heavily now. Though I wondered if he was really listening, I launched into an enthusiastic de-scription of what I had been up to. It took more than an hour to reach my mother's house, but I'd given up trying to tell my story long before then. It's hard to make yourself heard when your father is loudly cursing every other driver for his in-competence.

We pulled up in front of my mother's house.

"Well, in you go," he said, keeping the motor running.

I knew he had no more desire to stop the car and say hello to her than she had to come out and greet us. She didn't even want to let him in the front door. They had been separated for eleven years but were only now in the final divorce nego-tiations (a procedure that had outlasted several well-known

TV series). Although I did not have all the details—I didn't dare ask my father, and my mother never gave me the whole story—I understood that there had been a problem with the financial settlement.

He opened the trunk from inside the car, and I got out into the freezing air and retrieved my bag.

"Thanks a lot, Dad," I said through the window.

"I'll pick you up Thursday," he said, putting the car in gear, "for Hawaiian night at the golf club. I'll honk three times. Your brother and sister will be coming."

I picked up my suitcase (its mini-wheels powerless in three inches of snow) and made my way up the short path to the front door.

My mother lives in a three-bedroom beige split-level in a suburban development in the northwest of the city. This is not the house I grew up in, but it is full of my old things. It feels like home.

If you look east across the endless stream of fast-moving highway traffic, there is a strip mall whose occupants include Smiler's drugstore, the Treasure Chest (liquor), Bonapart's Pizza, Smash Video, a gas station, and a pub called Birmingham's, through whose doors I have never seen a single person enter or leave. Perhaps they are all locked in, drinking the place dry.

From my mother's back garden you can, on a clear day, see the silvery tops of the Rocky Mountains, one of my favorite places in the world. It takes about an hour to drive there, which is about how long it takes to get to the center of Calgary. Given the choice, I'll head for the mountains every time.

I rang the bell, waited a minute, and rang it a second time. The door opened soon after. I smelled warm cinnamon. She had been cooking.

"Mom—it's freezing out here!"

"Oh, sorry, dear," she said, giving me a hug. "I was just on the phone with Edna. She was having some problems with a new recipe and wanted me to walk her through it. Well, come in then. How was the flight?"

"Oh, fine, thanks. On time and everything," I said.

"Now, can I get you a cup of tea?"

"That would be great."

"And some apple crumble, hot out of the oven?"

"Terrific, thanks." My mother did make a great crumble. And having rejected the airline food, I craved something fresh and wholesome. And filling.

"With ice cream?"

"Sure, why not?" I could put the diet on hold for a few days.

We entered the sparkling kitchen, which she had recently refurbished with the help of her new boyfriend, Douglas. Now there were glossy modern cabinets, a hardwood floor, and an island in the middle for eating and storage.

"Very nice," I said.

"Oh, do you like it?" My mother's face glowed. "We finished just last week. Such a lot of work it was. And I pulled a muscle in my calf. But it was worth it."

"I'm impressed."

How could I not be? I didn't inherit my mother's domestic brilliance. A piece of self-assembly furniture usually had me in sobs after half an hour.

She served me some apple crumble and tea, and wiped the countertops as I ate. Mom was always in motion. Truth be told, we both found it difficult to just sit down and relax.

"Tina called earlier," she said.

Tina Miklechuk, an acquaintance from my last job, had

managed to avoid being downsized in the purge. In fact, she had been promoted to regional manager, which I could only put down to her relentless kissing up to the department head, a man who had brought on one of my migraines whenever he was nearby. She was now on her second maternity leave.

"I sent her an email to let her know I was coming," I said.

"She wants you to call."

"I'll call her back later," I said.

"She's such a nice girl and was upset that you haven't been in touch since you went to the big city."

"She hasn't called me, either," I said, trying to keep the edge out of my voice.

"She's very busy looking after those two kids of hers. They sound precious. I hope you'll have her over for a visit."

"That would be nice."

"Well, don't forget to call."

"I already said—"

"What?" My mother looked up from her wiping.

Breathe. It's too soon for a fight. Breathe! I'll call, I'll call. When I'm ready. If I ever am. Or maybe I won't. Just to drive you nuts, Mom. Oh, God, how childish. I've only been here ten minutes! All that work with Alan . . . Breathe . . . Smile!

"I definitely won't forget," I said, congratulating myself for my sweet tone. But that old feeling of being picked on was here again. And it was a hard one to ignore. How long would it be before I gave in to the temptation to return one of her verbal volleys with a backhand smash?

After a shower and a change of clothes, I went back to the kitchen to find that Mom had prepared her signature dinner: tuna pie and cauliflower cheese. She loves to cook, my mom, as well as being able to build a house from scratch. When she does her domestic thing, it always makes me feel inadequate, however—as I've said, I'm just not gifted in that area. Not that I haven't *tried* to improve. I was sent on my first cooking course when I was twelve, but all I can remember is throwing a saucepan of baked beans at a boy who was taunting me.

Over the years I've experimented with every cuisine known to man—but no man I've ever known has thanked me for it. My California rolls, my wholemeal loaves, my pumpernickel bagels, my chicken curries—none of them has won me more ardent admirers.

In my early twenties, while living in Montreal, I signed up for a yearlong cooking class at l'Académie Française de Haute Cuisine. I was instructed in the venerable art of French cooking by a man who had a small, waxed mustache and always wore a tuxedo. I learned the correct way to tie an apron (left over right, loop, right over left, double-loop), how to sharpen a knife with a granite grindstone from the Pyrenees, and how to julienne a carrot. M. Barbare—or Baba, as we came to know him—told the class that the word was first used in a 1722 book, *Le Cuisinier Royal,* and was derived from the technique of a famous French chef, Jean Julien. I mention this only because I have remembered the origin of the word *julienne* more clearly than I remember how to perform the act. But I did manage to master two French classics, *bisque de homard* and *coq au vin.* They'll certainly come in handy if I find myself having an affair with a French ambassador.

And I hadn't given up on my culinary education, either. Since coming to New York, I had enrolled in classes at a vegetarian cooking school and learned all about seitan and tempeh, which sound more exotic than they taste. Then I tested the durability of my relationship with Matthew by serving him up a meal that was so full of fiber he said he could have made a beach hut out of it.

So why have I gone to all this effort to become the queen of the kitchen? Not to impress men, not really: to impress my mother. And I have failed, not because I am a total klutz—although that's part of it—but because I have always rather enjoyed being the opposite of what my mother wants me to be. It's been like that since forever.

————

I was in bed and almost asleep when I heard a knock on the door.

"Katrina?"

Don't answer.

"Katrina? Are you asleep? It's Tina on the phone again. She wants to know why she hasn't heard from you. What do I tell her?"

I held my breath—the opposite of what I should have done in the circumstances—and tried to make myself disappear, the way I used to when I was a child. It still didn't work, but at last I heard her walk away. In the laundry room, the washing machine gurgled. It sounded like the damn thing was laughing at me.

When I woke up the next morning, Mom had already gone out. There was a note on the table.

Gone to Seniors Swimming Class at the Y. There's some leftover porridge with dried cranberries and walnuts on the stove if you're hungry. Tina Miklechuk: 389-4560. Don't forget to call. See you later. Love, Mom

I picked up the phone. It was now or never. And never was clearly out of the question while I was staying with my mother.

———

I was sitting in the window of the Bean There, Done That coffeehouse, which Tina had suggested for our meeting, watching the locals. This was one of the trendier spots in Calgary, and once upon a time I had thought it was very cool. Now it felt more like a retirement community. Across the way was Shear Heaven, the hairdressers; Scandals, the dress shop; Finnegan's Bake, the baker's; and Eternal Flame, the candle shop.

I stifled a smile.

Then Tina arrived, pushing a tandem stroller. I jumped up to open the door for her.

"Oh my God, Katrina, you don't know how lucky you are I'm here. Argyle threw up his breakfast—Argyle, say hello to Katrina, isn't he adorable?—and the other one in the backseat with the red eyes—she's just stopped bawling—is Paisley."

After we had rearranged half a dozen chairs and tables so that the tractor-size stroller could be placed out of the path of other customers, Tina fell backward into her chair and exhaled.

"I hope you don't mind, I'll have to feed Argyle in a moment. If I don't, he'll be impossible."

"Sure," I said. I just hoped she'd be discreet about it. "What would you like?"

"A weekend with Johnny Depp," she said. "If that's not on the menu, I'll have a double macchiato with whipped cream and chocolate syrup. And sprinkles. Thanks. And if you want to share something naughty, I won't object. Breast-feeding burns so many calories, I can eat anything. It's great!"

I went to order our drinks. And a chocolate chip cookie that was about the size of a manhole cover for $2 Canadian. Calgary may have had faults, but value for money was not one of them.

When I next looked, Tina had Argyle on her lap and was busy feeding him, while Paisley was burrowing under the table, eating what looked like crumbs. I hoped they were crumbs.

I set down the drinks. "Here we are," I said.

Argyle's head turned at the sound of my voice, and Tina's nipple sprang out at me, horribly red and engorged, as if accusing me of interrupting important work.

"Come on, Argyle, back on the job," Tina said. The little snapping turtle resumed his slurping, accompanied by rhythmic little gasps. "It's wonderful, being a mother. When are you going to try it?"

Before I could answer, Paisley stood up, reached over the tabletop, and grabbed the cookie.

"Not yours, sweetie," Tina said. "Let go, darling, let go." She gently tugged at the cookie, which broke into pieces. Paisley broke into tears. "Oh, God," Tina said. "She just won't stop today."

Then the little creature found a chunk of cookie on the floor and put it into her mouth. It wasn't our cookie, however.

"That'll keep her quiet for a bit," Tina said. "Now, tell me all about your new man. Has he proposed yet?"

"What, Matthew? I've only been living with him for a few months."

"Kevin proposed after four dates, but we both knew on the first that we'd be together forever. It's our fourth anniversary soon—where does the time go? *Paisley don't throw your cup on the floor I don't have another one. Pick it up there's a good girl.* You know that if it doesn't work out with Matthew there are plenty of guys here who'd jump at the chance. I saw Josh Pappas the other day, and he always had a thing for you. Carole—Carole from Human Resources, not the other one—told me that he is doing very well in real estate and looking to settle down. And she says he's had some body-work done—ab carving, it's all the rage here—and has a ripping six-pack. I'm not sure who told her or whether she saw it for herself. *Paisley I really mean it now stop that you are driving me crazy.* Oh, I'm having a barbecue Friday, if the snow's stopped. Josh'll be there. We're getting a keg, and I've invited loads of people from work—Havvy Ruffell from Accounts, Trish Moolers from Dispatch, and Johnny Paw-chik (you probably remember him as Johnny Tattoos, but he's had them lasered off). They all want to see you, so you must come. *Paisley put that down.*"

"Sounds great," I said. "I'll really try to make it."

"Now tell me everything you've been up to. What's life in New York really like?"

"Well, New York has changed me in so many ways," I said. "I've been doing yoga with a famous teacher and I feel—"

"*That does it Paisley you're going back in the car now young lady and Daddy will give you a good spanking when you get home.* Sorry, what were you—?"

"I was just saying that—"

But then the top of Paisley's sippy cup came off and she decided to empty the contents over my foot. Luckily, I was wearing snow boots.

"Oh God, I'm sorry," Tina said. "Look, the kids won't settle down and it's nearly their lunchtime so I had better get them home. Let's catch up on Friday at the party. The kids'll be at my mom's."

After Tina had left I sat with my coffee—untouched and now lukewarm—and tried to recover. I felt stunned by the flurry of noise and activity. And they weren't even my kids!

Matthew had once commented that anybody who wanted children had to be prepared to devote every minute of the day to them and to forget about any kind of quiet contemplative life. I had thought he was exaggerating wildly. But this little episode made me think again. Tina was in the grip of baby frenzy, and the capable woman I had once known was now the full-time, unpaid employee of her infants. And the mess! How would I cope with that, with my lack of domestic skills? This determination of mine to have children obviously required more clearheaded thinking than I had previously devoted to the matter. Did I have what I was now thinking of as the Three Qualifications for Motherhood: money, strength, and patience?

———

On Wednesday my friend Melissa, whom I've known since kindergarten, picked me up in her new Audi and took me out to a very civilized lunch, followed by shopping and a five o'clock martini. Although Melissa has two small children, she also has a very capable nanny. Very civilized, indeed. Perhaps motherhood could work for me, after all. But then I'd have to find a very successful husband like Melissa's.

I was fretting over how to excuse myself from Tina's Friday night barbecue, but in the end I didn't have to: it snowed so heavily in the morning that she called me to say it had been canceled. I did a wonderful job of sounding heartbroken. Too wonderful. Now she wants to come and visit me in New York. With Kevin, Paisley, and Argyle. I'm not sure the city can take the strain.

Hawaiian Night at the golf club lived up to its reputation, if not its name—piña coladas, which as far as I know are Mexican, were served. But we all enjoyed the time together: my sister awed me with a description of the open-heart surgery she had recently observed in medical school, my brother talked about his new job at an investment company, and my dad—well, my dad wanted our opinions on where he should go for his next vacation. And had brought the brochures.

After a week of trying to tell my New York story again and again to different people—married friends, work acquaintances, family—I realized that, for all the nods and smiles, nobody really thought of me as any different from the old Katrina. I began to wonder, in spite of *feeling* so different, whether I had changed at all. But then I reminded myself that this was Calgary, and everyone was seeing me through Calgary eyes. They didn't want a new and improved Katrina here at home; they wanted the Katrina they knew and approved of. So I decided to stop looking for my friends' and family's approval and just be me, whoever the heck that was now. *I* knew I had changed, and that was enough.

———

Then came the big test of my patience and restraint. It was bound to happen. I had been expecting it. Dreading it. And one evening, as my mother and I stood in the kitchen with cups of tea, and she related to me the minute-by-minute events of her day, it arrived.

"Well, what do you think?" She was tapping her foot.

"Mmm?" Apparently I'd missed something important.

"My new *shirt*? The one I was telling you about that I got from the charity shop for three dollars. Look."

I already had. It had almost given me retina failure.

"It's not exactly my taste," I said.

"What do you mean by that?"

"Bold-colored patterns. Not my thing."

"Well, if that's what you think," she said. "Not everyone can afford to dress like the models in your magazines, excuse me for saying so."

"I'm not being snide, Mom. It's just that I think you would look better in something more classic. You know?"

"Perhaps if you had had my life, you'd understand the true value of money, instead of throwing it about without a thought for tomorrow."

She turned and left me in the kitchen, and the next thing I heard was her bedroom door slamming. Not for the first time, it struck me how similar we were, how prone to harsh words, childish tantrums, hurt feelings. How it so often came down to *money*.

For a moment I stayed where I was, the familiar backwash of guilt for hurting my mother flooding over me.

I knocked on her door.

"Mom?"

No answer. I opened it slowly. She was lying on the bed, eyes closed.

"I'm sorry," I said.

She kept her eyes closed. I sat down on the edge of the bed.

"I said I'm sorry, Mom. Really. I don't always think before I speak."

She sat up. "Do you know how hard it was, growing up as one of nine other children?"

Uh-oh, we're off.

"I was the one they all turned to. I never had a moment's peace. No one ever thanked me for it. I gave up my youth to serve my family. I went to work at sixteen. You've had it easy, Katrina, compared to me."

"I know, Mom. I'm sorry."

"Sorry doesn't cut it anymore. If you don't like the way I dress, perhaps you should check out of my house and find a deluxe hotel, where you can admire the dress sense of the other guests. You treat this place like a hotel, anyway."

"Is that necessary, Mom?"

"You've always been so much trouble, Katrina. Right from the moment you were born."

"So you've told me on many occasions."

"The right side of my face went numb during pregnancy and stayed that way after the birth, and the pain from the forceps nearly did me in. But does anyone remember my suffering—or care?"

She brought her hands to her face.

"I know. I'm insensitive. Please forgive me."

I wanted to hug her. But I couldn't.

She took her hands away. "I never have this trouble with your brother or sister."

Zing! That did it. I got up off the bed.

"Perhaps if you treated me in the same way you do them, I'd behave more to your liking," I said.

"They don't feel the need to attack me the way you do."

"The way you attack *me*, you mean?"

"You only see things from your perspective."

How else was I meant to see them? I shrugged.

"And they show me respect," she said.

"And I suppose I don't."

"No, you don't," she said. "Please leave now, Katrina. I need to rest."

"Oh, Mom . . ."

And then, in a voice as icy and threatening as an approaching iceberg, she said: "Please respect my wishes, Katrina, while you're in my house."

I bit my lip. Why did it always have to come to this? *Why?*

———

As soon as I was sure my mother was asleep, I called Alan. He listened patiently—he had to, I hardly gave him time to speak—while I told him I felt fairly confident that I was about to lose my mind.

"My mom and I had the inevitable argument, and now I'm feeling guilty. I was trying so hard to avoid the old traps, but I fell into them just the same. She knows how to wind me up better than her old bedside alarm clock, and then, when I respond, she takes great offense—it's no fun for her if she doesn't get offended—and I have to apologize like mad. Then she goes cold and distant. And I have to spend a day or more trying to win her back—"

"Not so fast, Katrina, please! Start from the beginning."

"From the beginning? Okay, but I hope you don't have anything scheduled for the next few days."

"And can you speak up? I can hardly hear you."

I told Alan all about my relationship with my mother. How I felt that she favored my other two siblings and would always take their side. How she blamed me for the hurt I caused her during my teenage years without ever trying to understand how I had felt and how much I had suffered. And how we continued to pick at each other as if it were still 1987 and my wall was covered with Guns N' Roses.

"How did I ever end up in this family?" I asked him. "It's like we're from different planets."

"You may think you have nothing in common," he said, "but the yogis believe that each of us is born into the only family that we could have been. It was chosen for us by our spirit, before we were conceived."

Alan explained the yogic concept of *karma,* which literally translates as "action," and can be thought of as the seeds that motivate our spirit to enter into life. He said that I needed my family to fulfill my destiny, and that these relationships were vital to the formation of my character.

"You mean I *couldn't* have had a different family?" I said.

"Exactly that. Your family has been chosen to work out some of the lessons that you need to absorb during this lifetime."

"So things are never going to change between me and my mother?"

"Katrina, you must stop blaming your mother for the way your life has turned out."

"*Whaaat?* It's the other way round—she blames me!"

"But you are the one who must seek change."

"Why?"

"Because she is not going to unless you do. Be brave, Katrina, and show her the way. And if you need another reason, here it is: the longer you hold on to suffering, the more difficult it is to let go of."

It was like having a pail of cold water emptied over my head. I suddenly woke up to the truth. Alan was right. Wasn't he always?

At length I said, "I really do want to free myself from all the bitterness and ill feeling."

"And you will, Katrina, you will. Your intentions are good. Remember, you have everything you need inside."

I didn't want him to go, but he had another call waiting. We said goodbye and I hung up.

Then I crept to my room, lay down on the bed, and closed my eyes.

Alan's words rang in my head. *I was the one who had to change.* And I had to work out how for myself.

Before I had left for Calgary, Alan and I had been talking about personal relationships, and how hard it was sometimes to see the other person's point of view. He had introduced me to an exercise called the Equalizing Breath, which could be used to create the mental space to see the other person without the distortion (mindfuzz, he called it) that comes from being too close.

The idea of this breath is to create an inhalation and exhalation of equal length, which will symbolically erase the troubles of the past and restore equilibrium to the present, readjusting the relationship clock to zero so that you can begin afresh.

I was skeptical that I could pull this off without Alan's personal guidance, but as soon as I started the exercise, I could hear his voice again in my head as clearly as if he were sitting right next to me.

"Close your eyes and draw your awareness to the breath," I heard him say. "Breathe in and out through your nose. Notice the time you take to breathe in, and then try to breathe out for the same amount of time."

I spent a minute observing my breath, but I couldn't tell for sure if my breath *in* was equal to my breath *out*. This had happened the last time I tried it, and Alan had told me not to worry about the exact timing but simply to try breathing in and out evenly, making my breath as smooth and relaxed as possible.

"Surrender to the breath," he had said. "Don't force it or try too hard, otherwise your mind will become agitated, and negative thoughts will return to inhibit you."

He had previously suggested that I try counting as I breathed in and out, and when I felt confident my breaths were of equal length, that I cease all thinking—and just concentrate on feeling the evenness between my inhalation and exhalation.

The more I breathed, the more relaxed I became. All the tension I had felt as a result of the argument with my mother gradually faded away. I no longer felt resentment, blame, anger, or irritation toward her, or myself.

I let the breath bring me into the present moment, far from all the unwanted baggage of the past.

She was who she was. I was who I was. *You cannot change other people. You can only change yourself.*

The slate was clean. There was no winner or loser. I could only change the way I felt—and if I changed, it would no longer concern me whether or not my mother did, too.

———

The night before I was leaving Calgary my mother and I were in the kitchen. I was helping her to prepare a meal that would include Douglas, my sister and her boyfriend, my brother and his new girlfriend. She had given me the task of cutting the tops off the strawberries that were to go with the cake she had made for dessert. The only sound was the knife on the cutting board. I was taking my time to ensure that I removed the leaves without damaging the fruit. I wanted the result to look as pleasing as a photo shoot in her beloved *Martha Stewart Living*. It was all going so well when I heard a long, drawn-out sigh.

I looked up. "What's wrong?"

"Oh, nothing." She pretended to stir something in a saucepan.

"Then why the sigh?"

She turned to me. "It's just such a pity."

"What is?" I said.

"To cut off so much flesh with the leaves. You're losing half the fruit."

Without thinking, I took in my first breath, letting it out for an equal count before I replied.

"Well?" she said.

Her face was rigid with attention. She was looking forward to a final blowup before I left for New York. Something to feel miserable about until I came home for Christmas. When we could begin again.

I set down the knife. And smiled at her. And inhaled and exhaled again, making my breaths even. It was *working.*

I almost started to laugh. All these years she had been laying these traps and I had been falling into them. How stupid could I have been to waste all that time and energy on—what? On delaying my search for the truth about myself. This was not me. This endless round of sniping and retaliation—*it was not me!*

I did one more round of the Equalizing Breath.

"You know best, Mom," I said. "Show me how."

Breath Focus 6: EQUALIZING BREATH

Time: 5–20 minutes

Props: none

1. Stand, sit, or lie down. Close your eyes.

2. Take a few slow, deep, natural breaths through your nose. Allow yourself to simply observe your breath.

3. On your next inhalation, feel the entire circumference of your torso expand as your breath completely fills your lungs. Allow your pelvic floor, belly, and chest to expand all the way up through your collarbones.

4. On your next exhalation, feel all of the breath leaving your lungs as you release everything—collarbones, chest, belly, pelvic floor—back to the starting position.

5. Gradually extend your inhalation and your exhalation. Go slowly, breath by breath. Aim to equalize the inhalation and exhalation. If you can, make each breath slightly deeper than the one before.

6. At this point, if you are having trouble making the breaths of equal length, try counting. Start by inhaling for five counts and exhaling for five counts. Continue this breathing pattern for as long as you like. Feel free to lengthen or shorten the breath as needed. When you are comfortable, let go of the counting and just feel the consistency.

7. As it grows smoother and more even, notice how, when you become absorbed in the breath, space opens up in your mind, returning everything to equilibrium. See how the breath has brought you into the present moment, and how your perception of the world expands.

8. Let the breath create sufficient mental distance between you and the past to see yourself and the other person clearly, without the distortion of old experiences and memories.

9. Return to normal breathing.

A Note from Katrina

When I returned to New York, Alan and I had a long conversation about families. And he told me a bit about his own. It's quite a story.

His father fought in World War II with the Allies in North Africa and suffered from severe shell shock, which led to post-traumatic stress disorder. On his return to civilian life, unable to cope and with nowhere to go for help, he turned to drugs and alcohol to ease the pain. One of Alan's unhappiest memories was of finding his father passed out on the sidewalk in downtown Johannesburg. He had called his older brother, and the two of them carried their father home.

Alan's story made me feel a bit ashamed for having considered my own relatively normal family circumstances so distressing. In fact, the more I remembered the stories my friends had told me, the more I realized that we all face difficulties of one sort or another in our relationships with our families.

By practicing the Equalizing Breath, you will be able to see your personal relationships with what Alan calls *viveka*—a Sanskrit word meaning "clear vision." And with clarity will come compassion for yourself and others. You will no longer demand apologies or explanations. You won't need them.

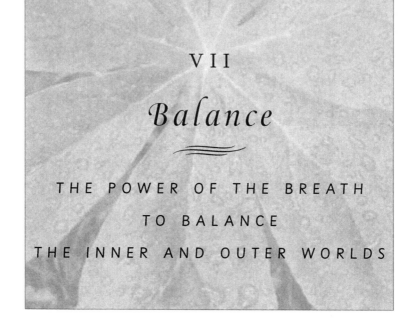

VII

Balance

THE POWER OF THE BREATH
TO BALANCE
THE INNER AND OUTER WORLDS

"YOU'RE A BUNCH OF PANTYWAIST WUSSES!"

Yeah? I'll show you, pal.

"IF THAT'S ALL YOU GOT GET YOUR ASS OUT OF MY CLASS!"

No way, I'd rather die.

"C'MON PEOPLE THIS IS RACE DAY NOT SLEEP-ALL-DAY!"

Okay, check this out, Spandex Man!

"GOOD, KATRINA, GOOD. YOU GO, GIRL!"

Spinning class. 0655 hours. I seemed to remember the beginning of a beautiful June day on the jog to the gym. Now I was in semidarkness, on a stationary bike, pedaling like a demented hamster, with seven other lunatics doing the same thing nearby. The only light in the room was coming from a disco ball hung from the ceiling. It was fever, all right, though not the Saturday night kind. I was soaked. And in the rush to get out of the house without waking Matthew, I'd rashly put on the pale blue bike shorts that show off a lovely, dark, sweaty V between my legs.

"OKAY PEOPLE NEARLY HOME NOW DON'T LET UP I'M WATCHING YOU PUSH IT PUSH IT GOOD NOW YOU GOT IT AWESOME AWESOME— That's it, you're done. Good job, people. Good job."

It's called Spinning because that's what my head does afterward.

At last my legs came to a stop. I felt weird. Was that the disco ball or were there lights flashing before my eyes?

"Katrina? Hey, lady! You okay?"

Jonas the Spinning Instructor was standing in front of me, his shaved chest glistening. His breath was garlicky. He had once announced, without anyone asking, that his favorite dish was octopus linguini. That might have explained it.

"You look a bit pale," he said.

"No kidding. I just did the Tour de France in forty-five minutes."

"Drink some water. Get something to eat."

"I'm fine," I said. *Although perhaps you could do something with my legs, I don't seem able to stand up on them.*

And then, out of the corner of my right eye, it looked like someone was waving a piece of tin foil.

Ah, no. Not now. Please.

Migraine attack.

Okay, no biggie, I've been here dozens of times before. I can handle it. I'll just walk slowly over to the wall to pick up my bag and wave goodbye to everyone and be on my merry way. Wherever that may be.

"Katrina?" Jonas again. "The door is over there."

Okay, so I got a bit lost. Easy to do when all you can see are a dozen flashing pinwheels.

When I emerged from the gym, the sun whacked me over the head with a giant yellow hammer.

I held my bag over my sweaty V, put one leg in front of the other, and marched home in a semistraight line while berating myself for not having listened to my body when it was giving me the warning signs—fuzziness, tiredness, sore eyes. I should have known that if I didn't rest I would end up like this, barely able to make it back to the apartment to collapse on the couch.

"What happened?"

I opened my eyes. Matthew was standing over me, looking concerned. I winced. Did he have to talk so loudly?

"Did you sneak off to Spinning again without telling me?"

I knew that, for the most part, Matthew admired my drive; it was a trait we shared. But it upset him when—time and again—I pushed beyond my limits.

"You don't look so well," he said, stroking my forehead.

"Can you please get me my pills? Massive migraine."

When I was strong enough to stand again, Matthew helped me into the shower; I washed, dried myself, and lay down on our bed. He drew the curtains, brought me an eye pillow, and softly massaged my temples. He was always very attentive when I felt ill, and I loved him for it.

"I've got a meeting with Alan this afternoon, and then writing class," I mumbled. "And afterwards I've been invited to a party by Romilly."

"You should cancel."

"But I want to go."

"Katrina, don't be silly. You're out of it."

"I'm going. I'll be fine."

"Why do you do this to yourself?"

Because if I exercise to exhaustion my mind goes blank and for a while I don't have to stress over anything, especially how insecure I feel about our future together. And when I get a migraine, you comfort me and then I know you must really care.

I shut my eyes. Was it really possible that I pushed myself so hard just to get a migraine so that I could feel better about our relationship?

———

When I opened my eyes again, Matthew was sitting on the bed. He handed me a cup of tea.

"How long?" I asked.

"Three hours."

I struggled to sit up and took a sip. I turned my head carefully in order to see the clock on the bedside table.

"It's only midday. I'm heading over to Alan," I said.

"I called and canceled while you were sleeping."

"You shouldn't have done that."

"Are you nuts? Do you want to make things worse?"

"Let's change the subject."

"Sure. Let's not talk about it. Let's not talk about any of the weird stuff."

My headache was flaring up again. Was I weird? Well, I did have screaming fits occasionally. And an obsession with counting calories. And counting in general. And then there were the Spinning classes, of course, and the whole headache thing. But still—

"What weird stuff?" I said.

"I was only joking."

"No, really. Tell me."

He sighed. "Forget it. I'm sorry."

I was too tired to think or talk anymore. I told Matthew I was going back to sleep again and asked him to wake me in two hours at the most. However awful I felt later, I was still determined to go to writing class and Romilly's party. Was that weird? Probably.

———

But I didn't leave the house again that day. The headache persisted until the early evening. I hadn't the energy to get dressed, let alone go out. I called Alan and made a new appointment for the next day, and left a message on Romilly's cell, apologizing for what she would soon discover was my absence from the party. I really couldn't face loud music or bright lights for at least another century. She probably wouldn't even notice, but I hate to let someone down.

After Matthew had made dinner for us, he sat down to watch a film, and I went to bed to read, but that didn't last long. The print was dancing before my eyes. I wanted to sleep, but certain nagging thoughts wouldn't let me. Was I giving myself migraines to make Matthew love me—or was it something more sinister? Supposing the reaction I was *really* hoping for was that he'd get so angry with me he'd *end* the relationship. Then I could run back to Calgary and forget about finding myself.

But I didn't want to leave Matthew. He was intelligent, kind, funny, and sensitive. I was attracted to him. And I thought the feeling was mutual. So why wouldn't he make a firm commitment to me? But did I *really* want to get married?

And was Matthew the right one, anyway? The whole situation was making me feel more and more confused.

I knew Alan was giving an evening lecture at the studio, so I impulsively called to get his advice. But it was Charlie who answered.

"Sorry, Katrina, he just left. Anything I can help with?"

"Oh, that's okay," I said. "I just wanted a chat with him."

"You don't sound so great," Charlie said. "Are you unwell?"

"Nothing a frontal lobotomy wouldn't cure."

"I don't advocate surgery," Charlie said, earnestly. "There are more holistic ways of curing the body's ills."

"Um, sure, Charlie." Then it occurred to me that she might have some advice about my migraines. So I asked her.

"You need some energy work," she said. "I know people who could help you. Are you free tomorrow?"

I hesitated. Knowing Charlie, the people she wanted to introduce me to might include an aura reader. But what did I have to lose? Perhaps there was an "alternative" solution to my problems.

I felt so much better in the morning that I almost forgot how rotten I had felt the night before. It's like that with migraines—somehow the agony is erased from the mind until the next time it comes on.

I opened the front door of the building to another beautiful summer morning: one of those perfect New York days that feature a cloudless blue sky, alpine-fresh air, and a sun that warms your face without sending you into a panic if you're not wearing SPF 30.

Charlie and I had agreed to meet at the entrance to Tompkins

Square Park on East Seventh Street and Avenue A. I found her sitting on a bench in lotus position, legs tucked up underneath. She was dressed in a flowing, silky summer dress, the kind of thing you might have seen in a documentary about the Summer of Love. She even had a flower in her long, dark, curly hair. Was it a chrysanthemum? Whatever, she looked great. Her eyes were closed as I approached.

"Charlie?"

Her eyes slowly opened. She had this dreamy look on her face.

"Hmm? Oh, Katrina. Hi. It's just so cool."

"What is?"

"Meditation, of course. I've been going really deep lately." She stood up. "It's great to see you!"

Charlie took my hand in hers. My first instinct was to pull it out again, but there was something in the innocent way she held it that stopped me. It was like the grip of a child.

"Your head feels better," she said, nodding. "I can tell. Yesterday on the phone I was getting a gray mist, but now I'm picking up bright orange."

She was talking about my aura, I guessed. Charlie had assumed that I was comfortable with the more exotic side of spirituality, but the jury was still out on that one. Not that I was going to say anything about my reservations. I didn't know her well enough to do that.

As we were leaving the park, we passed the dog run. Canines of every kind were kicking up a storm of wood chips and dust, barking and howling. Their owners seemed to be having as much fun as they were. I started to think that perhaps I'd persuade Matthew to get a dog. We could go for walks in nearby Washington Square Park—they had a splendid dog run there, too. If we could handle a dog, he might get over his fear of having a child. Then again, we didn't really have the room. And cats were out, alas—I'm allergic to cat fur. Perhaps a goldfish. But that would hardly convince him we could handle an infant.

Still holding my hand, Charlie led the way deep down into the Lower East Side, where she took me to visit a basement Chinese herb shop for the remedy *qiang huo sheng shi tang* (as big a mouthful to say as it was later to swallow), and then to a tiny, cramped shop selling crystals and jewelry made from semiprecious stones such as turquoise, agate, and jasper (known for their healing properties). The owner, a lady wearing an ill-fitting wig, was very talkative. I learned that the Druids had been the first space travelers, and how lapis lazuli could cure migraines. And she just happened to have—recently arrived—a charming necklace made from the same stone. At a special price. Encouraged by Charlie, I bought it, but I didn't think I'd ever wear it. Nor have I.

Then Charlie insisted on treating me to lunch, even though I told her I could spare only an hour before my appointment with Alan. She took me to a restaurant called Elixa, which served nothing but raw food, a trend that had recently become popular. She told me that she had given up all cooked foods, and that I should, too—eating raw made her feel amazing, like a goddess.

We were shown to a table and sat down. I studied her closely for goddesslike signs: her skin had an ashy pallor, and her teeth were a bit dull. Maybe it was the light in the restaurant. I tried to recall how she had looked before her new diet.

The waiter sauntered over. He was blond and very good-looking, and I was about to flash my whitened teeth at him when I saw he had black nail varnish. I went back to the menu. Before I could look properly, Charlie chose for me:

spaghetti made from bean sprouts with a cold nut sauce and, to drink, "young coconut" milk. We chatted briefly about life at the studio, and then the food arrived. We ate.

"Isn't it great?" she asked me, bean sprouts falling out of her mouth.

I nodded. It was ghastly, actually, but it made me feel much better about my own cooking. For dessert we shared a piece of raw almond cake. Until the moment I took the first bite, I had always loved cake. I began to think that, as a weight-loss method, the raw food diet was probably very successful—with every fresh mouthful I was being put off food altogether.

Then she said, "I'm glad you like it. People who don't are usually highly toxic individuals with a negative view of themselves and others."

"Is that right?" I said, almost gagging.

As we headed toward Alan's apartment, I began to think that Charlie might have hit on the truth. Perhaps I really *was* toxic. I felt a depression coming on.

"What's wrong?" Charlie asked. "You're frowning."

"Just thinking," I said.

"You think too much. Something I've noticed."

"That's my curse," I said.

"Well, I have a solution: stop. And *do* something instead. It always works for me."

"It's not quite that easy," I said.

"Yes it is. You just need to get more involved. I know—you love yoga, train to become a teacher."

Charlie was smiling and nodding rapidly. She seemed very excited by the idea. I wasn't so sure. Teach yoga? Get up in front of a class? Have people look at me, expecting me to be wise and graceful?

We had arrived at Alan's. I thanked Charlie for our morning together.

"Promise me you'll become a teacher," she said. "It's the right thing for you."

"I promise I'll think about it."

"No, Katrina, don't think—*do!* You'll make a brilliant teacher, trust me. Next time we go out I'll take you to meet Madame Ludmilla, who's the best tarot reader in the universe. I know she'll agree with me."

We hugged, and after a couple of minutes of that I pulled myself away as gently as I could. I watched Charlie cross the street and skip off into the crowd, a small but vivid figure in her flowery hippie dress.

In Calgary she would have been an oddity, but here in the East Village she was a natural fit. On the contrary, *I* was the one who felt out of place, with my suburban attitude. Charlie wasn't the one giving herself migraines: I was. And she might have been what my father would call kooky, but she also had a rare wisdom that came from being happy with who she was. I still had a long way to go before I could say the same thing.

I buzzed and Alan let me in. Fernando, his beloved Chihuahua, ran up to me and rubbed against my leg.

"I have to leave for an appointment," he said, "but while I'm away I'd like you to transcribe the lecture I gave over the weekend. The audio file is on the computer. And do make yourself some tea—you know where everything is. Is it all right with you if Fernando stays here while I'm out?"

"Of course, Alan."

I followed his advice and made myself a cup of jasmine tea. My stomach was feeling fragile after the raw food extravaganza, and I was glad to drink something that would help to settle it.

I put on the headphones and opened the file. The lecture was one that Alan had recently given to the trainee teachers on Tantric philosophy. It began by introducing the idea that the universe was created by the separation of two powerful forces that had once been joined together: Shiva and Shakti, the masculine and the feminine. Shiva represents all of the knowledge in the universe; Shakti is the source of all creative energy (we might call her Mother Nature).

I listened intently as Alan explained that our universe is made up of dualities, or opposites: light and dark, hot and cold, et cetera. For billions of years before our universe existed, these opposites were held in balance by the union of Shiva and Shakti. There was perfect harmony. But it was also a vacuum, and nothing could exist in it. To create our reality, Shakti had to separate from Shiva; this allowed man (and woman) to develop a consciousness through the world of the senses (hearing, sight, taste, touch, smell). But with these new powers came new restrictions: what the senses are able to perceive is only, according to Tantra, an illusion (*maya*).

Locked inside this illusion, we have lost the ability to connect with the higher spirit in ourselves and all things. The objective of Tantra is to transcend the sensory world and reconnect with the Divine.

I heard Alan's key in the lock and closed the file.

"Wow," I said, removing the headphones as he came in. "I really learned something from your lecture. I am completely caught up in the world of the senses."

Alan nodded. "We all are. It's hard not to be, when it presses in on us from all sides. Remember the bit about how, before the world was created, all the opposites were held in balance? Well, look what has happened since then. We live in a world of extremes. Look at the stark messages we receive every day from the media—you're thin, you're fat, you're gorgeous, you're ugly, you're rich, you're poor. How is anyone expected to see her path clearly when she is being pulled first one way, then the other? No wonder we lose our sense of balance."

"That's exactly how I feel—unbalanced," I said. "I always want to be *more*—better, thinner, fitter, sexier! It's a nightmare. I can never relax or take it easy. I always feel inadequate—a failure."

"That's what they want you to think, then you buy their products," Alan said.

I realized that my overdoing it at the gym was probably part of the same problem. I told Alan about my exercise habits, and my migraines.

"Of course it is part of the problem," Alan said. "Any excessive behavior is. The brain, as I'm sure you know, has a right and a left side. When our attention is drawn outward, one side of the brain dominates the other (you can tell which side is dominant by noticing which nostril is easier to breathe through). There is a technique I can teach you that alternates the breath between the nostrils as a way to balance the right and left sides of the brain. Using this technique will cure you of the tendency to lean too far one way or the other and indulge in extreme activities or self-judgments. Learn to balance the breath, I say, and you will learn to balance your life."

Alan's new exercise was called the Pendulum.

———

"This technique is one of the most powerful in the yogi's repertoire," he said. "By alternating the breaths between the nostrils, you draw your awareness inward. This helps to

regulate your emotions and your tendency to extreme thinking, and acts as an antidote to all the contradictory impulses
that pull you away from your inner truth. You will rediscover
your natural balance and harmony."

Alan instructed me to assume a comfortable cross-legged
sitting position on his rug, placing the backs of my hands on
my knees, with my hands closed in gentle fists.

"Feel your spine long and straight. Let your shoulders
relax. Then close your eyes and take a few moments just to
observe your breath."

I started to lengthen my breaths and grew instantly
calmer. It was amazing how, after these months of practice, I
could use my breath with ever greater ease to control what
was happening in my body.

"Now, the next time that you breathe in, open your right
fist and feel your breath moving into your right nostril," he
said. "This is a very subtle sensation, almost a thought. At
the end of the inhalation, close your right hand, and then
open your left fist and feel the breath moving out of the left
nostril."

This was a bit more complicated. I tried not to tense up.

"Keep your left hand open," Alan said, "and focus on
breathing in through your left nostril. Then close your left
hand, open your right fist, and breathe out through your
right nostril. You have just completed one round of the Pendulum. Continue breathing in through the right, out through
the left; in through the left, out through the right, opening
and closing the corresponding hands as you go."

I tried a few more rounds until I was confident that I
had it.

In through the right, opening the right fist.

Close the right hand.

Out through the left, opening the left fist.

Keep the left hand open and breathe in through the left nostril.

Close the left hand.

Breathe out through the right nostril, opening the right fist.

And repeat, starting with the right.

Alan told me that, once I had mastered the technique, I should try to even out my inhalations and exhalations. And after another minute I could really feel the side-to-side movement of the breath as it traveled in and out through alternating nostrils.

"I feel high. It's like I took some kind of mood-enhancing drug!"

"This is a very potent breath with amazing properties," Alan said. "We will practice six more rounds. As you breathe, the right and left sides of your brain are being harmonized. The headiness you feel now will give way to a remarkable sense of balance and order. Submit to the flow of the breath; it will do the work for you."

I did my six rounds. Occasionally I lost my rhythm, but gradually I found that the breathing was guiding me, instead of my having to guide it.

"Finish by breathing out through your right side, open your fists, and then bring the thumb and first finger of each hand together to make a circle. Remain sitting tall with your eyes closed. Explore the sensation."

I did. Maybe I was imagining it, but I felt different inside, as if my interior were a room in which all the furniture had been rearranged. Everything felt fresh and new. I did a mental pirouette around my new inner space.

"The breath is restoring your natural order," Alan added,

"and rejuvenating every cell of your being. You might sigh, or even yawn, while your body adjusts. And when the cycle is completed, your body will feel very still, almost *as though you were not breathing, but being breathed.*"

I sat in a meditative position for a few minutes, observing the effect of the exercise on my mind and body. I noticed that my head was not jumbled up with its usual contradictions. It felt like floating—inside. And when for a moment the peaceful emptiness was interrupted by a thought, I imagined that it was attached to the back of a small airplane, a fluttering far-off banner being pulled through the sky. It did not disturb my composure. And I felt a strange, gentle tingling all over my skin.

Softly, I heard Alan say, "Discover the wholeness at the core of your being. There are no pressures and no emotions. Nothing but empty space and tranquillity, the ambience of pure spirit. Sit for as long as possible in this state, so that your body can recharge and rebalance. Then, when you return to daily life, you will no longer find it necessary to go to extremes."

I sat for a few more minutes, oblivious of time passing.

From somewhere far away, I heard Alan's voice guiding me to place my hands together in front of my heart, as if for prayer, and to rub my palms together very gently. Then he had me separate my hands about an inch to feel the radiant energy between them. He directed me to bring my palms gently to my face and cover my eyes, and then to move my hands downward to the back of my neck, placing them there one on top of the other, and then one on top of the other at my throat, my heart, my navel, and my pubic line; finally, releasing the hands, to run them all the way down my legs to rest over the soles of my feet.

Then I bowed my head and slowly opened my eyes, first taking in a point on the floor in front of me, and gradually expanding my awareness to encompass the room.

I was alert yet calm, active yet relaxed, focused yet dreamy. Was this how a battery felt after charging overnight? Alan was right: the Pendulum was a very potent tool indeed.

I left his apartment feeling perfectly balanced on the inside and at ease with everything on the outside. As long as I could recapture this feeling whenever I needed it, I knew I would be happy just being myself and give up the allure of extreme thought or action.

Breath Focus 7: PENDULUM

Time: 5–20 minutes

Props: none

1. Sit in a comfortable cross-legged position. Place the backs of your hands on your knees and make gentle fists.

2. Lengthen your spine, relax your shoulders, close your eyes, and take a few moments to observe your breath.

3. Open your right fist, and as you inhale feel the breath moving into your right nostril.

4. At the end of the inhalation, close your right hand; open your left fist, and feel the breath moving out of your left nostril.

5. Keep your left hand open, and as you inhale feel the breath moving into the left nostril. Close your left hand, open your right fist, and exhale through your right nostril. This completes one round of the Pendulum. Begin a new round by breathing in through the right nostril.

6. Practice at least six rounds, more if your mind is particularly busy. Try to make the length of your breaths even. Feel yourself returning to the center (like a pendulum coming to rest), insulated from the outside world.

7. Finish by breathing out of the right nostril; keeping the backs of your hands on your knees, open both fists and lightly touch the thumb and first finger of each hand together to make a circle. Keep your eyes closed and sit in the stillness for five minutes, longer if you can. Try to absorb yourself completely in the experience, floating in spaciousness and feeling the wholeness at the core of your being.

8. Place your hands together in front of your heart as if for

prayer, and rub your palms very gently against each other. Then hold your hands about an inch apart and feel the radiant energy flowing between them.

9. Now bring up your palms gently to your face and cover your eyes, moving them downward to the back of your neck, placing them there one on top of the other, and then one on top of the other at your throat, your heart, your navel, and your pubic line; finally, releasing the hands, run them all the way down your legs to rest over the soles of your feet.

10. Bow your head and slowly open your eyes, first gazing at a point on the floor, then gradually expanding your awareness to take in the room.

A Note from Katrina

This is a technique that you could practice every day for the rest of your life to restore balance and internal order.

If you find it difficult to sit on the floor, you can sit in a chair with your back straight. At first, the coordination of the hands with the breath may seem a bit more complicated than our previous exercises, but please do not give up. A little application, and this breath will begin to show you some astonishing results.

As you become more adept, you will find that you need to do as few as one or two rounds in order to have the same mood-enhancing experience. The secret then is to learn to sit in the stillness afterward for as long as you can. According to Alan, one should try to remain seated for eighteen minutes after completing the exercise, in order to fully benefit from its healing and rejuvenation powers.

I often use the Pendulum when I feel I am becoming trapped in thoughts of an extreme nature; doing a few rounds calms me and, because it balances the right and left sides of the brain, allows me to move inward, away from self-judgments and limiting perceptions.

We live in the world of the senses, and they can lead us astray. It is all too easy to go to extremes of feeling and thought. The answer is to remember that it is all illusion, and the real truth is to be found on the inside.

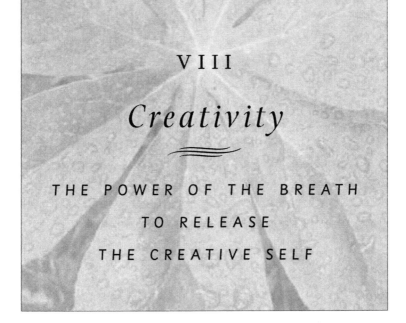

VIII

Creativity

THE POWER OF THE BREATH
TO RELEASE
THE CREATIVE SELF

"How's the writing going?"

"Matthew?"

I was so immersed in a fantasy I'd been enjoying (something to do with winning a National Book Award—the less said the better), I didn't hear him come in.

"Want to show me?" he said, dropping his bag and approaching.

Eek! I'd written only two lines the whole afternoon. I closed the document on my laptop in a hurry, knocking my teacup to the floor. Empty, thank goodness. Or he would have been on my case like Judge Judy.

"It's still a bit rough." I turned and gave him a bright smile.

"I could help, you know."

That was just what I didn't want. I closed the laptop. If I could have stuffed it under my T-shirt, I would have. Anything to stop him from seeing how little I'd done and wanting to interfere.

"I'll manage," I said. "But thanks for the offer."

"I'm here if you want me."

"I know," I said. "And I appreciate it."

What I didn't say was that I could not accept any more of his help. I had to do it on my own. I *had* to. Matthew's writing style wasn't mine, and whenever I let him look at stuff I had been working on, he offered suggestions that, however helpful, just weren't right for me. I had to find my own voice. But what *was* my voice? What made it different from other voices? And would anybody want to listen?

I just had this *feeling* that I had something interesting to say. But I didn't know how to turn the feeling into words. What was stopping me? It wasn't as if I didn't *want* to write. I did. Desperately. But almost as soon as I sat down at my laptop, I began to look around for something else to do. I surfed the Net. I made lists of things I would buy if I had the money. I daydreamed about being a successful author! How could I be a successful author if I never *finished* anything?

My writing class had now broken up for the summer. Without the camaraderie of my fellow students and Karen the teacher's friendly encouragement, I felt completely lost. Weirdly, I even missed Jennie the bike messenger. Not that she had shown me anything more cordial than a snarl the whole semester. My friend Lisa's theory was that Jennie's hostility was her way of showing that she was attracted to me. I had been a bit afraid of the tattooed lady all semester, but that thought absolutely terrified me.

Why did I need to be in a writing class to keep writing? Because, I realized, being in a group had made it easier for me to avoid having to confront myself with the truth: I was *afraid*. I was afraid of writing. No, that was wrong. I was afraid of *not* being able to write. I just had not been prepared for the agony of sitting in front of the laptop alone for hours at a time, waiting for inspiration to strike. The blank screen had become a wall I had to scale, rather than something to scribble words on.

So after many feeble attempts each day to write something good—and realizing with increasing desperation that it was all garbage—I usually abandoned ship in a near-suicidal depression and went out for a walk.

But doing that was hardly likely to improve my mood. Greenwich Village is one of New York's most creative neighborhoods, and going for a walk when you had just failed miserably to write even one good sentence was like wearing a sandwich board with THIS PERSON on the front and IS A CREATIVE FAILURE! on the back. I mean, you couldn't go a hundred feet without bumping into some blue wall plaque emblazoned with a famous name. On the other side of our street, across Fifth Avenue, was the club where the writer Samuel Beckett and the artist Marcel Duchamp had played chess; one street south of there was the former home of the poet Marianne Moore. The house that had been used for scenes in one of my favorite films, *The Hours,* was near our apartment (and Michael Cunningham, the author of the book, also lived in the area, so I had been told). Just around the corner, the Cedar Tavern had been *the* meeting place during the 1940s and '50s for artists such as Jackson Pollock and Willem de Kooning.

Even our building was a nest of creativity. The neighbors included two successful authors (fiction, cookbooks), a painter, a prize-winning poet, a prime-time comedy writer, a prominent stage actress, an advertising commercials producer, and . . . Well, I hadn't met the others. There was probably a Nobel Prize winner in 18B.

Matthew was rummaging around in the kitchen. If I left the desk, he might ask again about the writing. I decided against a walk and instead checked my email. I figured if he happened to come back into the room, it would at least look like I was typing. One new message from Romilly via her BlackBerry.

> Am in the Hamptons Thur-Tues til Sept. U will come. Love is all around. So is Big Money. R♥

I knew Alan was going to be out there in August, leading a teacher training. And although he'd sort of asked me to assist him for a fortnight, I hadn't had an official invitation. No way was I missing out on a summer visit to the Hamptons; it was a necessary part of my education as a New Yorker. I'd read that Puff Daddy, or P. Diddy, or whatever he was now calling himself, had bought a seafront estate and was converting it into a copy of the temple complex at Angkor Wat.

I was about to reply to Romilly when the phone rang.

"It's Alan. I have to go out of town to visit my son. Would you be willing to take Fernando overnight? I don't like to leave him alone for such a long time, and he knows you quite well now."

I told Alan I'd be happy to. Afterward it occurred to me that I should have asked Matthew first. I would just have to convince him. It was true that the apartment was too small for a dog, but Fernando was a very small dog, after all, and it was only for one night.

"Please, Matthew?" He was frowning. "Fernando's only a Chihuahua—he'd fit in an eggcup." Then I told him that I'd probably be away in the Hamptons for two weeks in August and he'd have the place to himself.

"Probably?" he said.

"If you let the dog in."

He agreed.

"So you're *glad* I'm going away for two weeks?" I said.

"It'll be a nice break for you."

"For you, you mean."

"Both of us."

He was smiling now at the thought of two whole weeks without me. I could quite happily be with Matthew around the clock, so I tried not to take it personally that he seemed to enjoy having his own space as much as (if not more than) he enjoyed being with me. I'd bet he was looking forward to renting Asian gangster films, eating cereal for dinner, and catching up on some *New York Review of Books* back issues that were in a neat stack awaiting his attention. At least I hoped that was what he was looking forward to doing, because even though things had been going well between us, and I trusted him, no woman leaves her unmarried partner alone for more than a couple of days without wondering what he might be getting up to.

So Alan came over and we all had a cup of tea and Fernando peed on the floor—but in the kitchen, thank heavens, which was tiled. If it had been on the living room carpet, Matthew's spleen would have burst. Even though it wasn't his carpet, and it dated back to 1972 or thereabouts, and had dark areas that looked like a weather map of approaching rain,

Matthew took care of it as if he had woven it himself. And he called *me* weird.

"I'll be back tomorrow afternoon around three," Alan said, handing me some prepared food for Fernando. "I am grateful to you, Katrina."

"You can always count on me," I said, hoping to plant the thought *HAMPTONS* in his head.

I looked down at Fernando, who was trembling even though it was eighty-five outside and the air-conditioning in the apartment wasn't working very well. Somehow he knew that his life was in my hands.

The poor pooch was so nervous at first that he couldn't stand up on his toothpick legs, and when Matthew and I took him out for a walk, we did the walking and carried him to Washington Square Park. I opened the gate to the dog run and gently set him down, preparing to undo his leash, but Fernando took one look at some of the beasts inside and started yipping and tugging me in the opposite direction. Being tugged by Fernando was like having your pinkie pulled by a baby. We settled for standing outside the fence and looking in at the romping dogs, which was all Fernando could stand in the way of excitement.

That night Fernando slept on the bed between us, curled up tight, his ears occasionally twitching as the night sounds from the traffic or the shouts of an inebriated reveler in the street interrupted his dreams of standing three miles high and stomping with giant paws on everyone below.

The next day I had planned to meet Lisa from my writing course at the Met. She was leaving for Vermont at the end of the week and would not be back in New York until September.

As much as I wanted to see her, in the morning I realized I'd have to cancel because of Fernando. I was about to call her when Matthew surprised me by saying he'd be happy to look after the dog for me.

"I didn't think you could handle a dog," I said.

"Did I ever say that?"

"No. I just assumed it." *Because you don't seem to want children.*

"I grew up with dogs. I love them."

"Really?"

"Sure. It's the dog hairs over everything that I can't stand. But I've noticed that Fernando doesn't shed. Have a good time at the Met. I'll walk him, don't worry."

If it is hot on the street, you can be sure that in the depths of Union Square Station it is positively thermonuclear. But there is no quicker way to travel uptown, and within half an hour I was at the foot of the broad stairway that leads up to the magnificent stone façade of the Metropolitan Museum of Art. People were sitting on the steps, enjoying the sun. I heard Lisa call my name and saw her about halfway up.

"How's the writing going?" I asked as we tried to enter the main hall through the throng of visitors.

"Not too well," she said. "I need some peace and quiet. When I get to Vermont, I plan to do nothing but write all morning and go hiking in the afternoon. I am determined to finish at least a couple of stories by the end of the summer."

A couple of stories? I'd be ecstatic if I could finish one.

"I'm so glad we decided to come today," I said. "I've been craving some inspiration."

Since I'd arrived in New York, I had visited the museum

at least a dozen times, but the thrill had not worn off. As soon as I entered the galleries, I was struck by the beauty and splendor of the artworks, and how *alive* they still seemed after so many centuries.

We wandered through the halls until we came to the Vermeer room. I wanted to show Lisa my favorite, *Young Woman with a Water Pitcher.*

"There she is," I said, easing us through a small cluster of Japanese tourists, who obligingly scattered. "See the way she has one hand on the pitcher, one on the latch, looking out of the window?" Lisa nodded. "Doesn't it seem like she is caught between the desire to go out and have fun, and having to stay in to do her tedious chores?"

Vermeer had somehow managed to capture exactly that moment. You could *feel* the tension in her pose.

"Amazing," Lisa said. "There's something so *true* there."

Lisa and I wandered the galleries for another hour, passing by one masterpiece after another. Again and again I marveled at each artist's unique way of seeing the world. That was what I wanted—to show the world that I had something to say. Something different. But how long would it be before I could honestly tell myself that what I wrote was original enough to be worth reading?

Suddenly I felt really depressed.

"Hey, I've had it," I said. "Let's get a drink."

We took the elevator up to the roof garden. There are few more glorious sights than Central Park seen from the roof of the Met. In summer the trees are swollen with dense green foliage, so full of themselves that they seem to be resting against one another for support.

I stared out over the vast green expanse and sipped my mineral water.

"Why do you write?" I asked Lisa after a while.

"For fun," she said. "If I'm never published, that's okay. As long as I can write for myself. It's another outlet for my creative urges. I play the guitar, too, did I tell you?"

"No! That's really cool." I envied Lisa's ability to be creative for creativity's sake. I often wished I could take writing less seriously. But I wanted more. At the same time, I wasn't at all confident that I had the talent. And I always got discouraged so quickly. Almost as soon as I started on a piece, I began thinking of reasons to stop. I could go on working as long as someone like Karen was watching over me, but as soon as I was on my own again, I just lost the will. Why was I always so stressed out when I was trying to write, and why was it always such a relief to stop? Why, when I wanted it so much?

A few years ago, in Canada, several girlfriends and I had been all fired up by a popular book of the moment that claimed to stimulate your creativity. We'd all followed it for a while and then, one by one, given up. It was just another fad book, after all. There was no magic spell to turn you into a writer. You could spend all your time reading about being creative—or you could just *be* creative. Which one was I?

It was time for me to think about getting home.

"I'll see you in the fall," I said to Lisa as we hugged on the steps outside the museum. We promised to send each other at least one finished story over the next month. I would miss her, my friend and ally in writing. I was dreading being alone in front of that screen again.

———

When I got home, there was no sign of Matthew or Fernando, but half an hour later they returned—with Alan. Alan and Matthew had met once before, when Matthew had come to pick me up at Alan's apartment, and they seemed to get on well together. Alan had told me that he thought Matthew was a "natural yogi" and a good guy.

"I got back sooner than I expected," Alan said. "Matthew and I took Fernando for a walk to the park. I just came back to thank you for looking after him. And to give you these flowers."

"Oh, Alan, that's so nice of you." They were beautiful. "Bring Fernando round any time. He's no trouble. Would you like a tea before you go?"

Matthew excused himself: there was a Tarkovsky festival at a nearby cinema and he had a date with some other guys from The New School.

"Pleasure talking with you," he said, shaking Alan's hand. He gave me a peck. "I'll see you later, love."

I brought out the tea, and Alan sat down on the sofa.

"Ah, you've been to the Met," he said, seeing the museum plan I had just put down on the coffee table.

"I went with a friend, Lisa," I said. "She's going to start coming to your class in the fall. We were looking for inspiration."

"Did you find it?"

"Not really. I mean, we saw amazing stuff, as always. But it's also a bit depressing, somehow. If you want to be an artist yourself, I mean."

"Why is that?"

"Because you see all these incredible, brilliant paintings, and then you compare your own pathetic efforts—"

"Why is it that a visit to the Met, when you enjoy it so much, causes you to feel bad about yourself?" Alan said.

I had to think about that one for a moment. Yes, *why?*

"I guess because I see greatness and know I can never be great myself."

Fernando looked up at me with moist eyes. I felt a bit like weeping, too.

"Don't you think *everyone* feels that way at the beginning?" Alan said.

He sounded disappointed. I had never heard that tone before. Was he losing faith in me? I couldn't bear that.

"Do you think Monet or Picasso did not have doubts at the beginning?" he continued. "Of course they did. What they understood—what *all* successful artists or writers understand—is that you must not be put off by opinions, your own or others'. You are too quick to come to conclusions. You must learn to give yourself a chance."

The one thing I have always found incredibly difficult is that if I don't get things right quickly—if people don't start praising me—I tend to give up. I explained this to Alan.

"There is only one solution: you must turn away from the outside world—from the need for approval and the fear of rejection—and look *inside*. You must enter your *own* world, the world of your mind. It is already filled with thoughts and memories, your childhood and growing up, your many experiences in life. It is a beautiful world, but it is only half alive until *you* inhabit it. Go there and find the answers to your creative dreams. But one thing above all you must have . . ."

I looked at Alan expectantly. Whatever it was—talent? ambition? strong typing fingers?—I was pretty sure I didn't have it.

"*Patience*. Patience, Katrina. It may take a year. It may take ten. You must write every day and wait for your time to come. And it will. I promise you—it will."

"But can I really write, Al? If it's going to take me ten years to be any good, I have to know."

"A writer is a seeker of truth. Can you find your truth by asking someone else? No. You must look inside, deep inside."

"But it's the uncertainty, the not knowing whether I'm on the right path—"

"The path will take care of itself. There is no map. Keep writing. Because, after all, what is the alternative?"

And suddenly I thought of the Vermeer again, and saw the truth of my writing problem. Like the young woman in the painting, I had opened the window—the window to creativity. But I was scared to look outside.

"I need help, Al. I can't do it on my own."

"That is the only way to do it, I'm afraid. But I may be able to point you in the right direction. I have another technique, something rather special, but I am not sure if you are ready to learn it yet."

"I am, Al. Really I am."

Alan looked at me closely for a few moments. Then he nodded.

"Very well. I will show you how to connect with the Unlimited Intelligence that exists beyond the mind."

Unlimited Intelligence?

"It is one of the most brilliant of yogic concepts," he said. "Imagine something that is invisible and imperceptible, for the simple reason that it is *everywhere*. It is here." Alan pointed first in one direction, then another. "And it is there." He pointed at my forehead. "Tap into the Unlimited Intelligence, and you can connect yourself to *the most powerful source of creative energy in the Universe.*"

Alan told me that the first step was to locate the pathway that would connect me with the Unlimited Intelligence, by exploring what he described as "the pause between two breaths." He explained that the pause between breaths is the moment between thoughts, which is where the door to Unlimited Intelligence lies. And what I would find beyond that door was *genius*.

"You mean I'll become incredibly clever and profound?" I asked. As if.

"The meaning of *genius* has changed over time," Alan said. "Like so many words that are used every day, it has been stripped of its original, more powerful meaning. When the word *genius* passed into the English language, some seven hundred years ago, it meant a guardian deity or spirit that watches over you from birth."

"Now wait a moment," I said. "Are you saying that's what I will find—?"

"What I am saying is that every great artist has made contact with the Unlimited Intelligence. It may have been by a different route from the one we will use, but he (or she) found it. It is the moment when you transcend the barriers of your own mind."

In order to begin the lesson, Alan explained the concept of *bandhas* (see the note at the end of the chapter). Then he asked me to sit comfortably and close my eyes.

"Start to pay attention to your breath," he said, "and focus on making it smooth, deep, and even."

This was easy enough by now. It took me no more than three rounds of inhalation and exhalation to become deeply relaxed.

"Now I want you to focus on the pauses in between the breaths."

I nodded. Or I thought I did. I already felt kind of spacey.

"Breathe in all the way, and then hold it in. Make it easier to retain the breath by drawing in your belly and pelvic floor, and letting your chin drop toward your chest, but keep your breastbone lifted. Hold for as long as you feel comfortable, and when you need to release, let your chin float back up as you exhale completely."

I continued to do this for about five minutes, sensing Alan's presence close at hand, although he did not speak.

And then he said: "Feel how still your mind becomes in the pauses between the breaths. And now, on the next pause, release yourself into the empty space and connect to the Unlimited Intelligence."

I wasn't sure exactly what I should do, but when I next inhaled and was holding in the breath, I just sort of let go of conscious thought . . .

. . . *and found myself drifting through nothingness. It was dark and yet not dark.*

If I had not already experienced the power of the breath, I would have opened my eyes in a panic and stopped whatever it was that was happening. But I felt calm. I felt free. I inhabited the emptiness without fear.

Somewhere in this endless space I heard Alan's voice:

"Enjoy the feeling of complete freedom that surrounds you. Be aware of my voice and not aware. Take your time. You have all the time in this world and beyond. You are being flooded with joy, peace, inspiration, intuition, and love. You are now a part of the genius of Unlimited Intelligence."

I continued to breathe, drawing further and further away from the earth and my own limitations—and closer to the truth.

"Dive into the pauses between the breaths. Hold a bit longer each time. Go deeper into the space. And deeper."

Trying to explain what happened then is difficult, but what I experienced was so astonishing that I hardly dared to believe it.

I was walking down a long corridor, at the end of which was a light and a half-open door. As I walked, I could hear voices. Sometimes I caught a glimpse of a face. Who were these people? I did not know. But I had a feeling of such warmth and love surrounding me. I continued to walk down the corridor. Someone said my name. That voice was joined by others until a great chorus was urging me on toward the door. Hands reached out to touch mine. And I felt so very peaceful. But who were these people? Why were they helping me? And now I stood before the door. All I had to do was open it and enter—

"Katrina?"

"Mmm?"

"Take a few normal breaths and then slowly open your eyes. That is enough for now."

As I did, a ray of sun suddenly shone through the living room blinds, dazzling me for a moment. A weakness came over me. I had to hold my head until I had recovered myself.

"Alan . . . I saw something. Witnessed something. I don't know . . ."

"Yes."

"A light. People. They were *there*, all around me."

"You experienced the Unlimited Intelligence."

"But who *were* those people? Guardian spirits?"

"Only you know the answer to that."

"But it's so confusing. I have to understand—"

"It will come to you. Everyone experiences the path to Unlimited Intelligence in a different way. All you need to know is that the connection is an experience beyond the mind. It defies description."

"It was so incredible, Al. I had this feeling of bliss, of oneness. Was I just imagining it?"

"Your experience with the Unlimited Intelligence does not require explanation, to yourself or anyone else. Believe in it, that is all."

I *did* believe what I had seen and felt. Somehow I had encountered the guardian spirits that had been attached to me from birth. They were the spirits of my creativity. I understood now what they were showing me—I *am* creative. I would never have to doubt it again. And I would continue to write, whatever the world thought of my work, because I wanted to, because I needed to, and because I *could*.

"Now I suggest you lie down and rest for a short while," Alan said. "And one more thing before I go—"

"Yes?"

"Do you still want to accompany me to the Hamptons for the teacher training next month?"

THE PAUSE BETWEEN TWO BREATHS

Time: 5–20 minutes

Props: none

1. Come into a comfortable seated position. Lengthen your spine and feel the crown of your head extending up toward the sky.

2. Close your eyes. Take a moment to notice your breath.

3. Start to draw out and deepen your breathing; try to make the inhalation and exhalation smooth and of equal length.

4. Inhale fully, and then pause and retain your breath for as long as is comfortable. As you hold the breath, draw in your belly and pelvic floor and drop your chin toward your chest to lengthen through the back of your neck. Keep your breastbone lifted.

5. When you need to release the breath, let your chin float back up and exhale completely.

6. Continue in the same vein: inhale fully; pause; exhale all the way. With each pause, see if you can hold a little longer than the time before, engaging your belly and pelvic floor and letting your chin drop down and your breastbone lift up to meet it.

7. Notice the space that is created in the pause and imagine yourself diving into that space. It is there that you can connect with your creativity. Don't try too hard. Just be receptive and open.

8. After fifteen to thirty breaths, let your breathing return to

normal, keeping your eyes closed. Take a few moments to observe the effects of your practice.

Do not attempt this breath until you have mastered the earlier ones. If, while doing it, you feel faint or disoriented, cease immediately, lie down, and breathe normally.

(Please note that pregnant women should *not* do this exercise.)

A Note from Katrina

Later, Alan explained that the pause between the breaths is called *antar kumbaka* in Sanskrit, and that the physical "locks" he had taught me are called *bandhas. Mula bandha,* the root lock that happens when you lift the pelvic floor, stabilizes your base and stops the outward flow of the senses. *Uddiyana bandha,* the drawing in of the navel, is also known as the "flying upward lock" and stokes the digestive fire as it draws energy up. *Jalandhara bandha,* dropping the chin to the chest, literally translates as "putting the lid on the pot" and keeps *prana* from escaping. All three locks facilitate breath retention and are vital to channeling subtle energy and concentrating it in your system.

I use this technique to connect with the Unlimited Intelligence whenever I need inspiration, and while I do not always have the same otherworldly experience I had that first day—it had probably been so powerful because Alan was sitting nearby, guiding me somehow—whenever I practice this breath, I become calmer and more able to enter a creative space beyond the limitations of my mind. I find it helpful to practice for five or ten minutes whenever I sit down to write.

Through this extraordinary breathing technique, Alan showed me how to create the space to let *genius* enter into my life.

Now it is your turn.

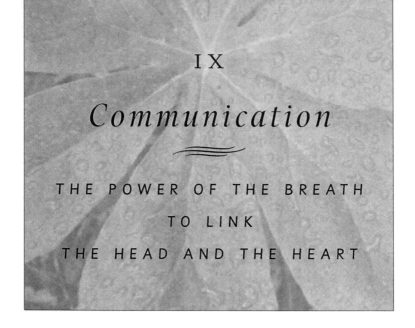

IX

Communication

THE POWER OF THE BREATH

TO LINK

THE HEAD AND THE HEART

"Katrina, is that you?"

Sky and sea had merged into one dense black backdrop, but I could make out Romilly's white shirt and long blond hair in the flickering firelight as she came toward me. I was sitting on a beach blanket with five other people, sipping a beer and discussing the property market. They were, anyway; I was only listening, or pretending to listen, while I pushed back my cuticles. Spread across the beach like an army encampment were other small groups lolling on blankets or posing around bonfires, drinking from cold bottles or silver flasks, examples of a type I could now identify with ease: Hamptons All-American (species: *Ralphus laurensis*).

"Romilly?" I stood up and brushed off some sand.

"Where've you been, K? I've been looking for you."

"Sorry—I was waiting for you."

"It's time to go. Come on."

We'd been guests at Skylar—heiress to an auto-parts fortune—Black's annual clambake on Georgica Beach in East Hampton. But the clambake, however compulsory, was only the appetizer to our main course, a party at the house-share that Romilly had taken for the summer with eight other people. Which might, I thought, explain her brisk tone: she was anxious to get to her bash, which she hoped would be talked about for the rest of the season.

The past week in the Hamptons had not been a disappointment. While Alan stayed with old friends who had a house in the Springs, I had the run of a three-bedroom, two-bathroom, one–games room "cottage" that belonged to one of Alan's regular yoga clients. I was now halfway through the two-week assistantship, and Alan was halfway through teaching the monthlong course for trainee teachers.

That weekend I had wanted to take the jitney back to Manhattan, but Romilly had insisted that I come to her party—"Please stay, I need support," she said—and when I tried to explain why I had to get back, she took my hands and said, "Look, just forget about Matthew for a minute, okay? There are going to be so many *amazing* people coming. Anyway, there's a heat wave this weekend and blackouts are expected in the city. It'll be a nightmare. You have to stay. You must stay. Pretty please?"

I could hardly refuse. Romilly treated me like an old friend, and I had to respond in kind.

In between trips to Barefoot Contessa for mixed-berry muffins and coffee, dips in Romilly's giant backyard pool, and a quick shop on Newtown Lane for something to wear that evening (a Michael Stars T-shirt was all I could afford, and that just barely), I had spent the day helping Romilly and her housemates with the preparations. A couple of hundred people were expected, and the party would be held outdoors to minimize the mess. The pool house had been transformed into a DJ sound station, five wet bars had been set up on the ample grounds, and several tents had been erected for the catering. The upstairs rooms in the house had been roped off, leaving the ground-floor kitchen and two bathrooms accessible.

Romilly had decided that she didn't want to arrive at her own do until it was in full swing, so we borrowed a brand-new silver BMW from one of her housemates and headed off to the clambake just as the valet parkers and DJ were arriving. Now it was nearly 11:00 P.M., and Romilly was eager to head back home—she planned to make the kind of inconspicuous entrance that the Pope does on Easter Sunday.

We drove for a couple of miles on dark, winding country lanes, and well before we arrived at her house I could see a long line of cars parked on the grass shoulder. One after another, gleaming in the hazy yellow of our headlights: BMW. Range Rover. BMW. BMW. Mercedes. Jaguar. Mercedes. Humvee. Mercedes. Range Rover. And on and on it went.

"I hope they've left us a spot in the driveway like I told them to," Romilly said.

"They" had. The valet captain pointed it out. We parked. Romilly checked herself in the rearview mirror. I opened my door—

"No, stop, wait. I need to prepare myself." She closed her eyes. "I'm beautiful. I'm fabulous. Everyone wants me. I speak Japanese. I'm a good person. I'm me me me me me."

She flung open the door and leaped out in the pair of seven-inch Jimmy Choos that she had just slipped on. Somehow she didn't stumble and break her knee on the gravel. I had to admire that.

"Tonight is our night." She turned to me. "Can you dig it, K?"

I nodded, smiling. She was high, she had to be—but on what I had no idea.

"No, I need to hear you. Can you *dig* it?"

"Yes."

"Louder."

"Yes!"

"Then let's get this party started!"

A bouncer working the door to the back of the house unlocked the gate for us, and we walked down the side path until we came to the largest house party I had ever seen. The pool was floodlit in rainbow colors, the music was loud enough to bring a bison to its knees, and women in slinky party dresses and Manolos were talking animatedly to men in button-down dress shirts, some of whom were also on cell phones or sending emails via BlackBerry. Everyone—man and woman—seemed to be over six feet tall.

When I looked around, Romilly had already been pulled into the vortex of partygoers.

"Hey babe—"

"Fabolus, you look fabolus—"

"This is so awesome *c'est un scandale*, Rom!"

I was left standing on my own. I did not know what to do. People zipped or floated by without a glance in my direction. I was underdressed, nobody knew me, and I had been abandoned. How long could I stand here before my fake smile sprained a cheek?

Relief arrived in the shape of Ben, a friend of one of Romilly's housemates; he was an investment banker who had grown up in Boston but was now the sole occupier of a town house that he had renovated himself on Manhattan's Upper East Side. Earlier, while I had been helping to prepare for the party, he had paid me quite a lot of attention, so I was pleased to see him again. We got drinks and chatted for a while about Martha Stewart's sexual orientation. He had the nicest manners and the best shoes, and I found him quite attractive. Which made me feel guilty. I always feel guilty when I am getting on well with a man other than my boyfriend. I blame this on my mother and the time she marched me to the manager's office at the local Safeway to apologize when, at age three, I unthinkingly took a stick of candy from the bulk bin. Thanks to Mom, I feel the need to confess if I so much as *think* about being dishonest. And flirting with another male when you have a boyfriend is uncomfortably similar to sneaking candy from a bin.

So I told him about Matthew. But Ben remained just as attentive once he found out—perhaps even more so—to the point where I began to wonder if he was actually interested in me. Not that I wanted him to be, but I kept thinking back to the conversation Matthew and I had had before I left and wondering whether, perhaps, I should start looking more seriously at other men.

Then he told me I looked like a young Catherine Deneuve.

I blushed. "I do? That's very—"

"No, not Catherine Deneuve. Rene Russo."

"Rene Russo?" *Well, that's okay, I guess.*

"No, sorry, not her—"

"Who?" I said. *Rhea Perlman?*

"I can't think of her name at the moment. She was in an ad for a whitening toothpaste. Do you bleach your teeth? They're so white. Anyway, I think you're really attractive."

"Thanks." He *was* hitting on me.

"And, honestly, if I wasn't gay I'd be all over you."

Eh? How had my gaydar missed *that*?

For a moment I felt let down, then relieved. Now I could forget about whether I would or should or could let him kiss me and just have a good time.

Ben did what gay guys do best for girls: he squired me around for the rest of the night, introducing me to hedge fund managers, LBO specialists, M & A experts, arbitrageurs, and a host of other acronyms and titles that left me bewildered and awed. They all had girlfriends who were models, or looked like models. Or at least dressed the way I imagined models dressed. In between these introductions, and glasses of champagne, Ben brought me up to date with all the celebrity news I had missed by being away from my laundry room.

The party wound down as dawn was rising on the horizon, and when I asked Romilly if I could help with the cleaning up, she told me not to be silly, they'd hired a crew to do all that.

While we were taking off our makeup before bed, we talked about the party. She was happy with the way it had gone, and there had been a photographer from *The East Hampton Star,* so pictures of it would be in the next issue. Sometimes these pictures were picked up by trendier magazines looking for summer news, and Romilly was hoping that she might be seen in *New York* magazine or *Interview.*

"So many men hit on me," she said, "I couldn't keep track of the number of times I gave out my number."

"You give it out to just anyone?" I asked.

"Sure. I love getting phone calls. And if I can't remember who it is, or it's someone I can't stand, I just say no."

Then Romilly asked me if any of the men I had met appealed to me.

"I'm with Matthew, Rom, remember?"

"It's just that Ronald Hass asked about you."

"Oh? Who's he?"

"Only one of the richest guys at the party. But that shouldn't be of interest to you, you're happily taken."

I nodded.

"He asked for your number."

My heart sped up a bit. That was bad.

"I hope you didn't give it to him," I said.

"Of course I did. At least let him meet you, he'll never forgive me otherwise. And if you don't, *I'll* never forgive *you*. This could be your big opportunity."

I had trouble falling asleep. I didn't want to go out with Ronald Hass. But things weren't that simple now. Before I had left New York for the Hamptons, I had given Matthew an ultimatum.

"I need to know whether we are going to stay together," I had said.

"We'll be together for as long as we're both happy," he replied.

"But that doesn't make me feel secure," I said.

"Security comes from knowing that the two of us are happy, not from some piece of paper calling you my wife."

"That's not very reassuring, you know."

"Look," he said. "Are you happy now?"

"Yes."

"Then what's the problem? Neither of us can tell how

happy we'll be with each other a year from now, or longer."
He looked at me. He shrugged. "Can we?"

That's not the point, I wanted to say. How can I be happy
with a man who won't guarantee that he'll stay with me?

"I'm sorry, Matthew," I said. My adrenaline surged and I
felt almost sick. "That's just not good enough anymore.
We've been together almost a year. If you can't offer me a
better sign of your commitment to this relationship, we'll
have to end it. I'll be in the Hamptons for two weeks. I'd like
your answer when I get back."

We left it at that. I didn't know whether it was a good sign
that he had chosen not to argue with me then and there. Perhaps he had already made up his mind. Perhaps we were already finished. And perhaps I should not reject the idea of
Ronald Hass out of hand.

———

The morning after the party, Romilly and I rolled downstairs
for a late breakfast before she and her housemate Jasmine,
whose car we had borrowed the night before, headed back to
the city. The plan had been for Rom to take the jitney on her
own—Jasmine and her fiancé, 'Van, were planning to be in
the Hamptons for all of August—but now Jaz, a partner in a
PR firm, had been called back into the city for a few days
because her major client was having a crisis, something to do
with a babysitter.

"It's such a pain," Jaz was saying. "We were supposed to
go to a lunch my friend is hosting in Montauk today, and
now 'Van has to go alone. He hates arriving anywhere without a woman on his arm." She stirred her coffee and gave
me a thoughtful look. "But I have an idea. Katrina, if you
don't have any plans this afternoon, why don't you go with

him? 'Van is great company. I'd hate him to be disappointed."

At that moment 'Van entered the kitchen. Without asking me, Jaz told him what she proposed.

"Great," 'Van said. He ran a hand through his thick chestnut hair. "I can show you Montauk," he said to me, "and drop you back at your place later."

"Sounds fun," I said without thinking. I had the day to myself and did want to see Montauk, which is at the easternmost tip of Long Island. "But I won't know anyone."

"No problemo," said 'Van. "You're safe with me. I'll introduce you around."

A few hours later, 'Van and I were sitting in his antique convertible Porsche; we passed through Amagansett and then followed Montauk Highway along the coast. It was a stunning drive, and the wind in my hair gave me a feeling of freedom that I found unexpectedly intense and exhilarating. So what if Matthew and I split up? It didn't mean I would have to go back to Calgary. I could make a life for myself in New York. I felt sure I could do it with Alan's support, and now that Romilly had taken me under her wing, I would not lack for social events.

'Van and I talked about his relationship—"Jaz is great, we've been together for six years." His job—"I basically just focus on making money, and I'm very good at it." His car—"I bought it at this great boutique car dealership in Tribeca; it's the same kind that James Dean had." We didn't talk much about me, but I was okay with that; I was more interested in hearing about his platinum lifestyle than in telling him about my own more mundane kind.

And then he said, "I hope you don't mind, but you're not pronouncing my name correctly."

"Oh, I'm sorry," I said. "What am I doing wrong?"

"Well, it's *'Van,* not Van."

"I don't think I—"

"Look, before you say the *V,* just take a quick breath. Like ha-Van. See what I mean? Ha-Van. Sort of like a gulp. Try it."

"Sure," I said. "Uh-Van."

"Almost."

We arrived at his friend's house, and I was glad I came; the lunch was delicious—lobster salad, corn on the cob, sorbet. 'Van was attentive to me, and so his friends were, too. I relaxed and had fun. Afterward, as promised, he took me on a tour to Gosman's Dock and the famous Montauk Point Lighthouse. The weather was so clear that we could see Connecticut and Rhode Island, and we decided to sit on a bench for a few minutes in the sun before heading home. I had closed my eyes and was enjoying the sensation of a light breeze on my face when I felt an arm snake its way around my shoulders.

"What are you doing?" I said, sitting up with a start.

"Don't tell me you can't feel the vibe between us," 'Van said.

Oh no. Had I given off the wrong signals? I wondered if I could outrun him to the only house I could see, a mile or so away on the headland. I imagined pounding on the door and shouting for help while 'Van laughed maniacally behind me—"Make all the noise you want, this house has been empty all summer, and there isn't a living soul for five miles!"

I shook my head to clear it. "Listen, 'Van," I said, "you have a girlfriend—"

"Who, *Jaz?* She's cool."

"And I have a boyfriend."

"What's he got to do with it?" 'Van said.

I stood up. "You're great, and I'm flattered—but no, thanks."

His face was turning red.

"I'd better get home now," I said.

We didn't say another word to each other during the drive back to the house. He pulled into Lily Pond Lane and parked. 'Van just stared straight ahead, his hands tight on the wheel. For a moment I thought he was going to hit me. Then he flicked the unlock switch. As I was getting out of the car, he said, "Let's just keep this between us."

"No problemo," I replied.

———

I spent the rest of Sunday under a pink and blue striped umbrella, lazing on a chaise longue. Once in a while I jumped in the pool, which I had been told I could use whenever I wanted. I didn't see Alan's client, the film director, or any of his family. The book Matthew had recommended to me, *My Ántonia*, lay unopened on the grass. I was too spent to concentrate. But I couldn't stop obsessing about the conversation I'd had with Matthew before I left. I ran it through my mind again and again. I loved him. And I really believed he loved me. Why had I given him a silly ultimatum? Why?

I had to talk to him. I dialed our number. No answer.

In the evening I had a bowl of cereal and watched *Sex and the City*. The episode seemed particularly frivolous and absurd. I called Matthew again and again. No answer. I thought about calling Alan, but I didn't have the number at the house where he was staying, and he always turned off his cell phone on the weekend to get some peace.

I went to bed with a knot in my stomach, convinced that Matthew was already gone.

———

Monday morning. The birds woke me at four. I went for a swim. How delicious and somehow sinful it was to jump into a warm pool in the semidarkness. A totally empty, perfectly kept, completely private pool. The sun came up. I drank orange juice and made myself a peanut-butter sandwich. Thought about Matthew. Dialed the number. Still no answer. There was only one possible reason: he had spent the night with another woman. I knew there was someone at The New School who had been after him; she had called several times but never left her name if I answered the phone.

Just after seven, Alan picked me up to take me to the training, which was being held in a church hall near the Windmill, an East Hampton landmark. We arrived to find the trainees in groups, chattering, warming up, or sitting cross-legged on the floor, studying cue cards with pictures of yoga poses. The hall was high-ceilinged and drafty, but the sun had already begun to shine through the skylights, and once the training started it would not be long before hoodies and leg warmers could be safely removed. Today the trainees would begin to practice teaching each other *asanas,* the postures that constitute the physical practice of Hatha yoga.

As soon as Alan walked in, the energy level went up a notch and the trainees became more bubbly. They crowded around him, excited and enthusiastic. He spent some time chatting amiably with them and drinking the tea that one of the trainees had bought for him in town.

When everyone had settled down, the morning class began. Alan gave a talk about the physical practice of yoga, explaining the meaning of the word *Hatha,* which is composed of the syllables *ha* (sun) and *tha* (moon). Learning this, I was again reminded of how yoga often combines two opposites to make a whole.

"Just as the sun heats and the moon cools," Alan explained, "the yoga postures are meant to strengthen and energize areas of weakness, as well as stretch and relax areas that are too tight. Hatha yoga is about finding balance, and each *asana* requires careful attention. You must bring awareness to the functioning of your muscles and the alignment of your body, while continuing to focus on the breath."

Then he led us through a sequence of poses, and after that the teacher trainees started to work with each other.

The training went well and finished in the late afternoon. Instead of going straight home, I decided to take a walk to a nearby beach. I sat on the lip of a sand dune, looking out to sea. The sun sent ripples of silver light over the water. Two seagulls, like puppets on invisible strings, were swaying to and fro a few feet above the surface of the sea, riding the air currents. I tried to concentrate on the soothing sound of the waves softly breaking on the shore, but my mind was agitated.

"I was told that I might find you here."

I turned, shielding my eyes from the glare.

"Alan? Oh, hi. I was a million miles away."

"May I join you for a moment? It was so stuffy inside the hall."

"Please."

For a while we sat in silence, just looking out to sea.

"Is there anything wrong?" Alan asked.

"Wrong?"

"You seem rather reserved today. Not your usual self."

"I do? I'm sorry. I've been thinking about whether or not I have a future with Matthew. Love is such a pain."

The sun had gone behind some clouds. The sea turned from blue to pale green.

"Did you know I have been married?" Alan asked.

I shook my head.

"Twice. And neither time did I ever expect to get a divorce. But people change, and things do not always turn out the way we expect them to. That is why it is so important that you discover your own truth, and not settle for someone else's. Now, what's going on between you and Matthew?"

As usual, Alan got straight down to business.

"He just won't commit to the relationship. Before I left New York, I gave him an ultimatum: either he makes a commitment to me, or it's over."

"Do you really think that giving Matthew an ultimatum— even if he accepts it—will ensure a lasting relationship?"

"No, not really. But that's what I've been told I should do."

"By whom?"

"Friends." Romilly, for one. Tina from Calgary. Even Lisa seemed to think it was a good idea. I always asked other people for their opinions about my problems and then listened to their advice over my own instincts. I had no faith in my ability to do the right thing for myself.

"So you wouldn't have issued this ultimatum unless you had been advised by others to do so?"

I shook my head. "I'm just so afraid that one day he'll tell me it's over."

I felt in my heart that Matthew loved me, but my head was

giving me a conflicting opinion. My friends were all of the "no ice, no dice" persuasion, but truth be told I would be happy without a giant rock on my finger. One carat would do. Or even a simple band dotted with smaller gems. No, even that was more than I needed. As long as I knew that Matthew wanted a future with me, I would be quite happy to forgo the bling altogether.

"All my life I've made decisions without knowing why I'm making them," I said. "And then I second-guess myself and ask if I did the right thing. It's like my head and my heart are at odds with each other."

"Then it is appropriate that we are here at this moment, because I can show you a breath I call the Ocean Breath," Alan said. "Just as the tide moves back and forth across the shore, constantly changing the boundary between earth and sea, so the Ocean Breath acts as the intermediary between our head and heart, bringing us to a greater understanding of who we truly are and what we really want."

Alan went on to explain the power of the Ocean Breath. The throat, which plays a major role in this breathing technique, is situated between the heart, the center of a person's individual consciousness (*jiva atman*), and the head, where the Universal Consciousness (*param atman*) resides.

When the throat center is purified and balanced by the Ocean Breath, it facilitates communication between *jiva atman* and *param atman*. This allows the individual's consciousness to bloom, achieving the state of *jiva mukti* (living liberated). When you are liberated, you can communicate truthfully with yourself and others.

Alan taught me this lesson with the two of us side by side on the sand, looking out to sea.

———

"This breath is audible," Alan said. "Done properly, it makes a sound similar to the ocean. The vocal cords are narrowed slightly while you inhale and exhale, allowing the sound to ebb and flow, like the sea washing over the sand."

I thought of how soothing I found the sound of the surf, and how healing it was to be near the water.

I learned that the Ocean Breath has three qualities. First, it compels you to focus on the sound, which teaches you to listen more closely to yourself. Second, it slows down the breath, which eliminates distractions and creates the space inside you for the head and heart to make a connection. Third, similar to the ocean washing the shore, the breath sweeps away limiting judgments and belief patterns so that you can be more receptive to yourself and others.

"The easiest way I have found to teach the breath is to start with the mouth open," Alan said. "So please begin by inhaling and retaining the breath. Then place one hand in front of your open mouth, about three inches away, with the palm facing you. As you exhale, breathe onto your hand, as though fogging a mirror or a pair of glasses. It sounds like *haaaa*."

Alan told me to draw out the exhalation. The breath felt warm and moist on my hand. Then he said, "Now please inhale with your mouth still open, and this time try to imagine fogging a mirror *behind* your head, making a sound more like *ahhhh*. You can even place a hand there, if it helps."

I exhaled with my hand in front of me, as I had done before, and then I moved it behind my head as I breathed in, while imagining a mirror behind my head. I did this a few times, inhaling and exhaling through my mouth, until I was comfortable with the *haaaa* and *ahhhh* sounds.

"Stage one completed," Alan said. "Now please *close* your mouth and try to get the same feeling as you breathe in and out through your nose. Close your eyes, too, if you like. Don't force the breath; just let it caress the back of your throat, and it will make the sound of the sea breaking on the shore. One . . . two . . . one . . . two . . . Gently, gently. Feel your breath slow down as you listen ever more closely to it. Pay attention to all of its subtleties."

———

When we had finished the exercise, Alan and I just sat together for a while. The sun was starting its slow descent toward the horizon.

"I must be getting back," Alan said. "Can I give you a lift home?"

"That would be great," I said. "And thanks for teaching me the Ocean Breath. I feel so much calmer and clearer. I already had serious doubts about whether I did the right thing with Matthew. Now I am sure of it. It was wrong of me to force him into a corner."

"That reminds me," Alan said. "I've been meaning to tell you the subject of our conversation that afternoon we took Fernando for a walk in Washington Square Park."

"Oh?"

"It was you. And I received the strong impression from Matthew that he is very committed to the relationship."

I nodded. "I think I knew that all along," I said. I had never seen anything to make me believe otherwise. Why couldn't I trust my own eyes?

"Matthew has been cautious," Alan continued, "not because he does not care for you but because he wanted to see how much you cared for him. As I see it, he has given you support and understanding while you make the transition to your new self."

Now I felt ashamed of my behavior. I hoped it was not too late to rectify it.

"I'll call him as soon as I get home," I said. I could only pray that this time he would be there to answer the phone.

Breath Focus 9: OCEAN BREATH

Time: 5–20 minutes

Props: none

1. Come into a comfortable cross-legged seated position.

2. Inhale and place one hand three inches in front of your face with your palm facing you. Now, feel the muscles at the back of your throat constrict, and with your mouth open exhale onto your hand as if it is a mirror you are trying to fog (you will make a *haaaa* sound). Feel how the breath is warm and slightly moist.

3. Then imagine that you have a mirror behind your head (bring your palm to the back of your head, if this helps). As you inhale through an open mouth, imagine fogging the mirror *behind* you, feeling the same constriction at the back of the throat as you did when you exhaled (see step 2). This time the breath will sound more like *ahhhh*.

4. Once you have successfully created the sound in the throat, it is time to transfer the breath to the nostrils. Retain the same feeling of fogging the mirror, but *close your mouth and breathe in and out through your nose.* If you find this challenging, start each inhale and exhale with the mouth open, and halfway through the breath, close your mouth.

5. Without forcing the breath, pay attention to its sound. Feel the back of your throat narrowing as you breathe in and out. Close your eyes if you like.

6. Keep your focus on the breath. Feel it slow down and deepen. Let yourself be fully present. Just listen.

A Note from Katrina

The Ocean Breath acts as the intermediary between our mind and soul, uniting the passion of the heart with the logic of the head, and bringing us to a greater understanding of who we truly are and what we want from life.

Practice this new breath every day for several weeks until it feels comfortable. It is not difficult to do, but it can take a little getting used to (especially the odd new *haaaa* and *ahhhh* sounds you will hear).

This breath has taught me how to get in touch with and respond to my true self. Gradually, the gap between feeling and thinking is narrowing; the two parts of my consciousness, head and heart, are being joined together fluidly and responsively—like sea and shore. And now that I can better communicate with myself, I can communicate so much better with other people. I have begun to really listen to what I am saying, and to what is being said. At last I am truly present when I make a decision. Above all, I have learned, communication is not about *making* someone understand you, it is about *being understanding*. And to be understanding of others, we first have to understand ourselves. This breath will go a long way toward attaining that goal.

Do give the Ocean Breath time to work; you will discover that it changes you in subtle ways that you do not notice at first, rather like the ocean's effect on the shoreline. Before too long, you might find that you are another big step closer to the person you have always wanted to be.

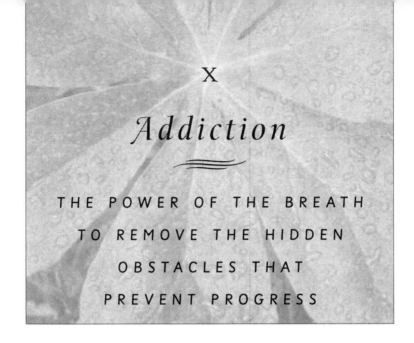

X

Addiction

THE POWER OF THE BREATH
TO REMOVE THE HIDDEN
OBSTACLES THAT
PREVENT PROGRESS

I called home several times before I returned to New York, but each time there was no answer. If I had not been busy helping Alan with the teacher training, my anxiety would have been uncontrollable. Instead I diligently practiced my breathing exercises and tried to balance the danger signals coming from my head with the trust I had for Matthew in my heart. I loved him; he loved me. Everything was going to be fine.

And it was. It really was. Right up until I arrived home on Friday evening to find an empty apartment. There was an envelope on the table marked KATRINA. Scenes from films with letters on tables flashed before me. Farewell letters. Farewell forever letters.

I opened the envelope as slowly as I could, trying to stay calm. The contents were not as bad as I had feared. Not good, but not disastrous. Matthew had gone to Philadelphia to stay with his friend Mark the screenwriter in the house Mark had recently inherited from an uncle. That autumn Mark was teaching a screenwriting course at Penn and had invited Matthew to attend as his guest. Matthew wrote: "Mark has plenty of room and he thinks the course would be useful for my writing. If I decide to stay, it means I will not be returning to New York until Christmas."

And that was all. Was he leaving me? It didn't look like he had made up his mind. Yet. There was no address on the letter, no number at which to call him, and Matthew didn't use a cell phone. I'd been cut off.

I spent Saturday in a daze, trying to read between the lines in Matthew's letter. He hadn't told me to leave his apartment, but he hadn't told me to stay, either. He'd be back at Christmas, he said. That was almost four months away. Did he expect me to sit in his apartment until then, not knowing if we were still together?

And then that evening he called.

"Can we just forget what happened before I left?" I said.

"I don't know." He had that dry-leaf tone to his voice.

"I made a mistake. I'm sorry," I said.

"I've got some thinking to do."

"Do you love me or not?"

"I thought I did."

"Well, I love you," I said.

"People who love each other don't issue ultimatums."

"I panicked. I don't want to lose you."

"Let's talk later," he said. And put down the phone before I could ask for his number there.

———

I fell asleep on the couch, staring at the phone, willing it to ring. He didn't call back. I woke up again at 4:30 with a frightful headache. I dragged myself to the bed and fell on it. Now I couldn't sleep. I had the whole bed to myself, something I'd been looking forward to for months, because it was so small and uneven that when the two of us were in it you had to lie perfectly still or bump the other every time you turned over. And all I could think was: *I wish Matthew were here, holding me. Telling me I am forgiven.*

When I awoke, it was to a perfect day. Sun. Blue sky. The weather was positively Mediterranean. I thought I should go outside and take a walk, only I didn't want to leave the apartment in case Matthew called. But would he? I felt panic rising up like brushfire, and there was nothing I could do until it was raging out of control. I was going to lose my boyfriend. And it was my fault. Totally and utterly my fault. All my life I have shied away from blame. I'll do anything to escape it. Well, this time there was no escape. I couldn't invent an excuse that sounded plausible. Even to me.

I made myself some tea, and then I resumed my vigil, sitting on the couch, staring at the phone. I had to talk to someone. I called Alan.

"What do you think I should do?" I asked him.

"What do *you* think you should do?" he replied.

"I don't know, Alan. I'm not thinking very clearly at the moment."

"Then do nothing. It was impatience that caused you to

issue Matthew an ultimatum in the first place. Don't make matters worse. What will happen, will happen."

Do *nothing?* No, no, no. My mind was like a mosaic that had been smashed to pieces—thoughts were scattered everywhere like marble chips. I had to do *something.* I turned on the laptop and tried writing. I stopped. This was impossible.

The phone was ringing. Matthew?

"Hello?"

A female voice, as smooth and efficient as a tightly tucked-in hotel sheet: "Ms. Repka? I have Ronald Hass on the line for you."

Ronald Ha—? OMG.

"Katrina?" There was some interference on the line. "Is that Katrina?"

"Yes it is."

"I'm in Switzerland. Calling from the top of the Jungfrau. That's some four thousand meters above sea level. The snow is the purest white I have ever seen."

"Um, what are you doing up there?" I said.

"Well, I'm about to—no, I *am*—skiing down."

There was more interference—

"Can you still hear me?"

"Yes," I said.

"Thank goodness for Bluetooth. Look, I won't keep you; I think I'll need to focus on the descent for a while. But I'll be back in NY on Wednesday. May I see you?"

No. Yes. No. Yes.

"I don't know," I said.

"Good. My driver will pick you up at six-thirty Thursday evening. We have tickets for the Kirov, and then I hope you'll join me for a light supper. Looking forward to it. *Auf Wiedersehen!*"

The line went dead.

Was Ronald really skiing down the Jungfrau? Even if he wasn't, you had to admire the presentation. And if he was, then wow. Matthew didn't ski. He didn't drive. And he wasn't here. It may have been superficial of me, but the desolation I had been feeling as a result of his absence was swiftly replaced with irritation, if not anger. So he didn't want to talk to me? Fine. Someone else did. Someone pretty amazing, it seemed. I wasn't going to stay in the apartment feeling lonely and unloved.

I went to the kitchen to make myself another cup of tea and begin a series of interlinked fantasies: ballet—dinner—diamond necklace—private jet to the Seychelles—wedding on the beach—Frank Gehry apartment downtown—

And my cell rang. *Don't answer it,* I thought, *it's Ronald canceling. He mistook me for some other female. Easy to do from the top of the Jungfrau, four thousand meters above sea level.*

"Well? What did I tell you?"

"Romilly?"

"Wait till you see his Warhols. He's been buying up modern art as fast as his dealer can sell it to him. He says that everything will be worth ten times what he paid for it in five years—"

"Romilly, I've been meaning to ask—"

"No, I haven't. He's just a friend."

"What do I do about Matthew?"

"Sorry, K, can't talk now. I'm late for my lunch date."

———

On Monday morning I told myself I had to attend to the backlog of errands, emails, and Alan-related tasks that had piled up while I was away in the Hamptons. Not that I wasn't grateful for the distraction. It meant I could stop mulling over what I should do about Matthew. Or what I was about to do with Ronald. But Thursday came so quickly I didn't have time to talk myself out of the date with him.

At 6:30 on the nose, the buzzer of the apartment rang and I went downstairs. I knew I wouldn't be walking very far, and I had dared to put on the new, slightly-heeled shoes that I had bought on sale at Barneys Co-op, which matched my favorite shirt from Agnès B. I had debated whether or not to put on the one skirt in my closet, but in the end decided on jeans. I had never dressed up to go to the ballet before, and I didn't want to feel—or look—as if I was trying too hard.

Ronald's driver was waiting for me on the sidewalk and led me over to a black Bentley with tinted windows that he had double-parked (like Alan, he seemed unruffled by the cars honking behind him and drivers shouting threats out of their windows). He introduced himself as Ash, Mr. Hass's personal driver. The back door opened with a *whoosh* like the door to a bank vault, and I slid into the creamy leathered interior. The door closed. Absolute silence. It was so damn comfortable that sitting up seemed like a waste—I wanted to roll around on the softness like a baby on a blanket. Now a hint of music—something Cuban—wafted through the air as the car moved off and away. There was as much room here as in our bedroom, I swear.

I began to fret again that I had underdressed for the ballet. Or even for the car. Then I reminded myself that I didn't want Ronald to like me too much, and if the jeans turned him off it might be a blessing.

After a few minutes I began to feel the need to speak to someone to calm my nerves. I pulled out my cell and dialed Romilly.

"I'm in Ronald Hass's car en route to Lincoln Center."

"Nice one, K," Romilly said. "Now remember the mantra: you're fabulous, you're gorgeous, you're you."

I didn't feel much like me in the back of this chariot.

"I'm still feeling guilty about Matthew," I said.

"You're having a night out, you're not eloping," Romilly said. "Or are you?" She chuckled. "I expect a full report in the morning, if it's not already on Page Six of the *New York Post*."

"Hey, how did that lunch date go——?"

But Romilly had already gone. She did not have time for chitchat.

The car was now passing through Times Square; how I loved the blinking lights, the milling crowds. All the plays and musicals Matthew had taken me to. How much fun we had had. I couldn't do this—I couldn't. I leaned forward to ask the driver to turn back. No, that was silly. I wasn't going to let anything happen with Ronald. And it never hurt to make a new friend.

"Mr. Hass is waiting for you in front of the fountain," Ash the driver said, when we pulled into the drop-off area. And sure enough, I could see him from the top of the steps when I entered the plaza. He was wearing a business suit: probably just left the office. More handsome than I remembered, too, and tall (and dark—he was so tanned he looked like he had spent a month in the Caribbean. Which no doubt he recently had).

"How good of you to come," he said, kissing me on both cheeks. Thanks to my time spent in Montreal, I was able to execute this maneuver with the confidence of a true *jeune parisienne*, who kisses the air rather than the face—although I couldn't help but notice his smooth shave and clean smell. He'd taken some trouble.

"Thank you for inviting me," I said. "I'm so excited to be seeing the Kirov."

"Should be worth it," Ronald said, "although it's better to see them in St. Petersburg. The program is Balanchine, by the way."

"Are you a big fan of dance?" I asked.

"My mother was a ballerina. Shall we go in? The performance will begin soon."

Ronald led me to our seats: orchestra, front and center. I usually sit in the nosebleed section. It was a real treat to have a close, unobscured view of the stage, especially because I wouldn't have to pull out my glasses. Not that I thought I looked bad in them. But, you know.

The performance was spectacular, and during the intermission Ronald took me for a cocktail to the members-only lounge, where he told me more about his childhood.

"I grew up here in Manhattan," he said, "on Central Park West, just around the corner from the Museum of Natural History. My mother still lives there. I went to school in the city and then to Yale to study applied mathematics. After that I received an MBA from Stanford. But it never occurred to me to leave New York permanently. This is my home. London is fun, Paris is elegant, Tokyo is a trip. But New York is all of that—and more."

After the performance he suggested dinner at Babbo on Waverly Place. I had wanted to get a reservation there forever, but it is more difficult than long division. You have to call the restaurant a month to the day before you want to go, within the first half hour of opening. Usually the line is busy, or you are left on hold for ages. The one time I finally got through, most of the reservations were taken, but they could offer me a table at 10:30 P.M. I declined. Only Argentineans eat at that hour.

"Don't we need a reservation?" I said.

"They are expecting us." Ronald smiled gently. Of course they were.

Ash the driver was in the same spot I had left him, and the drive downtown was smooth and fast. Going south in the evening, you can often do ten blocks before the lights go red. Ash drove so skillfully it was like being inside a video game. He dropped us outside the converted town house in under fifteen minutes.

As soon as Ronald entered, a great fuss was made over him, and then we were ushered upstairs to our table. The wine list was presented. The sommelier whispered in his ear. Ronald chose a vintage Barolo. It was opened with a grand flourish and poured into a decanter. I felt high just on the fumes. And I had never tasted anything like it. Rich, smooth, mysterious. It traveled down to my belly with a delicious lack of haste, lighting up every bit of me as it went.

We spent the next couple of hours talking about life, art, and our common interests, which ranged from skiing to the novels of Edith Wharton. The more we spoke, the more relaxed I became, but I hardly touched the food. Not only was he successful but he was very interesting and, on the surface at least, a decent guy. We got on well.

"Do come back to my place for a drink," he said. His credit card lay on top of the bill. I tried not to look. But what kind of card was that—titanium? Uranium? "I'm only a few minutes away."

It was, as they say, crunch time. But the Barolo had worked its spell on me. And, I confess, I was curious to see where he lived. As any girl would be.

The car was outside, of course. In less than ten minutes we had arrived a mile or so farther downtown, at Ronald's loft apartment in a building on North Moore Street in Tribeca.

And it was amazing. Huge windows. High ceilings. On one side, views of the Woolworth Building; on the other, the Empire State Building. There was no clutter. Everything was hidden behind vast sliding doors. The decor was steel, wood, and white paint. It was the ultimate minimalist pad.

I saw two Warhols on one wall. There was a large stone sculpture in one corner. Henry Moore? It might have been.

Ronald selected a bottle from the stainless steel wine storage unit and poured me a glass. While he changed out of his suit into jeans, I checked out his CD collection. Many of my favorite bands were there. Then I took a seat on what could only have been a Mies van der Rohe Barcelona daybed. An original, I assumed, not a copy.

"I shouldn't stay too long," I said, as Ronald emerged from his bedroom at the other end of the loft. "I have to meet a friend at yoga in the morning."

"Ash will take you back whenever you are ready," he said.

But I wasn't ready. Yet. We talked for another hour or so, and I stole a glance at my watch—midnight—and was about to suggest that I really ought to leave now, if only so that Ash could get to his own bed, when I found myself locked in an embrace. And enjoying it. Quite a lot. Too much.

I pulled away. (Not immediately, you understand.)

"Ronald, I had a great time this evening," I said. "But I do have to get up early."

I stood up. Ronald nodded and stood up, too.

"Of course. I'm off to Hong Kong tomorrow, but I'd like to call you when I get back. Perhaps you'd come and visit me at my house in the Hamptons."

"That sounds lovely," I said.

Ash dropped me home at around 1:00 A.M. My head was fuzzy from the wine and my lips were tingling from the kisses. I picked up the phone. Messages.

9:00 P.M.: Hey, it's Matthew. I'll try later.

10:00 P.M.: It's Matthew again. I tried your cell: it's off. Hope you're having a good time.

11:15 P.M.: No message.

12:02 P.M.: No message.

12:53 P.M.: I hope he's worth it.

Feelings of guilt and shame—feelings I hadn't had for so long, thanks to Alan and my breathing exercises—rose up inside me, flooding me. But it was only a *date,* nothing serious. I tried to calm myself. Breathe, *breathe.* No chance. I lay down and curled myself up into the fetal position, which only reminded me that now I would never have a child with Matthew. I hadn't meant to break up our relationship. *I hadn't meant to!* I wanted to call Alan, but it was too late. And I couldn't, anyway. He didn't deserve to hear any more of my foolishness. He'd *told* me to be patient. Why hadn't I listened? But it wasn't *serious* with Ronald. I was just feeling lonely and unloved.

I'd ruined everything.

I got up. Went to the kitchen. The light outside was pearly gray. I shivered. Made myself a coffee. My head hurt. I felt a bit sick—but more than that, I noticed, I felt hungry. *Unimaginably hungry.* I looked in the fridge. Nothing. Matthew and I never stocked up; there was no need to, we ate out most of the time. I wrenched open the freezer: Ben & Jerry's Chunky Monkey. I'd forgotten all about that. *Oh, you little darling, come to Mama.* But wait—I didn't want the sugar yet. That would come later. What I wanted now was . . . pizza.

Pizza.

Now *that* was what I wanted. The biggest, cheesiest, greasiest, sickliest pizza I had ever ordered. I wanted to eat until there was no more room left in my body, until my fingers were swollen and every pore of my skin was oozing hydrogenated fats. *I've destroyed our relationship.* Only food could help me now—help me forget, soften the landing at the bottom of the pit into which I was free-falling. Eat. Eat. Eat. Eat. *Eat.*

I opened the kitchen drawer. Where was that leaflet? The twenty-four-hour pizza place. Still there. "Papa Angelo's. Serving the Village Since 1947." I dialed. Please answer. Please.

"Do you have a pizza big enough for four people? Good. I want one. With double cheese, mushrooms, pepperoni, garlic. And a large bottle of Coke. Not diet. It's free with the order? Even better. And please hurry. We're hungry."

I lay down on the couch to await its arrival. This was the old feeling, the good feeling. Food didn't let you down. People did.

———

It all started at the age of eleven. That was when I discovered the gorgeous, slim, out-of-this-world models in magazines. Under their spell I stopped eating, almost, and lost twenty pounds in a matter of months. *This is awesome.* But I was always hungry. A couple of my friends were dallying with anorexia, but that was no good. I wanted to eat. I wanted to eat the whole world. Then one day I was at my school friend Aimee's house, and she told me that she had a little secret. I watched while she ate an entire box of Oreo cookies and a pint of Dreyer's strawberry ice cream. Then she took my hand and led me to the bathroom. There, doubled over the toilet bowl, she threw it all up. *Ugh, I don't like it. But Katrina it means you can eat whatever you want and NEVER GET FAT.* So later I tried it for myself. And after I had thrown up I felt so relaxed, so numb. My body was empty. My mind was empty. From then on, for a few brief moments, from four to nine times a day, I would lie on the floor by the toilet and feel completely blissful and at peace. Nothing could touch me. No one could touch me. I was free. I had bulimia. I had bulimia. Bulimia had me.

———

I lay on the couch and sweated. It would be here soon. *Food.*

My thoughts drifted back once more to that grotesque period in my life. It was all a terrible mistake. My parents couldn't begin to understand what was happening, and it frightened them. So they sent me off to dieticians, doctors, and counselors. *I don't want your help. I don't want to talk about it. Leave me alone!* I became the bane of the family, the subject of hushed phone calls and the object less and less of parental concern and more and more of parental resentment. *I make your lives hell?* I wanted to ask them. *What about my life? Do you know how I feel?*

It was here.

I could smell the pizza before the delivery guy had touched the front door. The stench of hot dough and grease. I overtipped. *Don't tell anybody—it's our secret.* I was shaking as I opened the lid. The surface was still bubbling. *You done good, Papa Angelo, you done real good.*

The first slice gave me such a jolt of pleasure I could only liken it to the feeling a heroin addict must get after receiving a much delayed fix. I chewed three or four times and swallowed.

The second and then third slices passed through almost as quickly. I was a conveyor belt, a machine for mastication. Saliva exploded in my mouth. Hot fat ran down my chin. I pulled another slice from the box, the cheese slipping off one side; I coiled it around a finger and thrust it into my mouth. After the third slice, I was more than full. But I was racing now, racing downhill, I was skiing to the finish. On my own personal Jungfrau. I couldn't—I didn't want to—stop.

There were eight broad, glistening slices. I ate them all. Then I wiped my face with a towel and started on the Chunky Monkey. I turned on the TV, some infomercial. I watched it avidly, spooning ice cream automatically into a freezing mouth that a few minutes before had been burning hot. Laugh or cry? I still wasn't sure.

At last it was over. I lay back on the sofa. My belly seethed and heaved. Now I would go to the bathroom, bend over the toilet bowl, and send it all back to hell, where it came from. Just as I used to do.

No. I mustn't let myself.

"Alan?"

"Katr— What time is it?"

"Six-thirty. I'm sorry. There's no one else I can talk to. I need your help. I'm in trouble."

"Come over, then. I'll have the tea ready."

I dressed as quickly as I could, swallowing again and again to stop myself from throwing up. I wouldn't give in. I'd fight this. Alan would help me.

I half ran, half walked over to Alan's place. He let me in immediately.

"Oh, Alan," I said, bursting into tears as he opened the door, "I've been so stupid."

He talked me down, as I knew he would. I spent the next few hours asleep on his couch.

———

It was Sunday afternoon, two days after my breakdown. Alan and I were meeting to travel together upstate, where he was giving a workshop. He had been asked to talk on the *chakras* (the seven energy centers) to a group of yoga teachers. My task was to tape the lecture and transcribe it later for future reference.

Leaning against a shady wall outside the East Village parking garage where Alan kept his car, I pulled out the latest *New Yorker* magazine from my bag. I had just finished skimming the cartoons—always hilarious—when I heard a familiar buzzing sound. Looking up, I saw Alan in a loose white shirt and jeans, zooming toward me on his electric scooter, hair flying in the wind, big smile on his face. People were turning to catch a glimpse of him—not an easy thing to get people to do downtown, home of everything trendy and attention-grabbing.

He pulled up beside me, and the scooter ceased its buzzing.

"Hey, Al."

We hugged.

"How are you?"

"Better," I said. "Much better. I owe you my life."

"What?"

"For the other day. I really thought I was going over the edge."

"All I did was sit down and talk to you. I don't deserve any medals for that. Come on, let's get the car."

The attendant conjured up the Land Rover from the dark, and Alan folded his scooter and put it in the back. We were soon heading uptown on First Avenue, stopping briefly to pick up chai lattes, after which we would cross the Triborough Bridge and leave the city behind.

"Tell me more about your eating problem," Alan said. "We didn't really talk about it the other morning."

For the next hour I gave Alan the full story. How my bulimia had started as an innocent game and ended as Russian roulette. How I wasn't equipped to understand the deeper feelings behind what I was doing: the insecurity, the unhappiness, the loneliness, the anger.

And now, nearly ten years later, it was back. Matthew's absence, the uncertainty of when or if he planned to return, my guilt at going out with another man, not to mention the large amount of wine I had consumed . . . "I guess it all brought on the attack," I said. "I've tried so hard to cure myself, but this addiction is like a part of me that I can't shed. Not just a part of me—sometimes I think it *is* me, the real me. God, I'm pathetic."

"The first stage of your cure must be to stop calling yourself names. Or condemning yourself in any way. I have told you this before. You *must* pay attention to the words you use. They are powerful weapons that can do you a lot of damage."

I nodded.

"Perhaps you still have this eating disorder because you have never completely transcended the forces that are the cause of the problem. Addictions are insidious, because they cannot be treated from the outside. Addiction to food cannot be cured by dieting. Addiction to alcohol cannot be cured by abstaining. It is our *unconscious* that governs this aspect of our being, not our conscious mind. And the unconscious is exactly what it says—something we have no awareness of.

We think we know ourselves, but our needs and drives are concealed far under the surface, where, just like a volcano, they occasionally erupt and cause havoc. There are still deeply buried conflicts inside you that can trigger the onset of bulimia. To be truly free, you need to remove the roots of the problem."

"If only I could," I said. "But I think my addiction may be stronger than my will to get rid of it. It's like some evil demon inside me."

"People often use words like *demon* to describe an addiction," Alan said. "And that's quite understandable. An addiction does seem like a curse, something wicked or evil. The problem, however, is that this 'evil' is also a part of us. So we end up by hating *ourselves* when we cannot get rid of it. And that's very sad."

"Sad and complicated. I don't understand how it got such a hold on me."

"You don't need to," Alan said. "We can leave those questions to the psychoanalysts. What we must do is simply release you from the destructive, negative patterns that are deeply and tightly entangled in your unconscious. According to yogic philosophy, your unconscious mind is housed in the lower part of your body. That is where we must work, on the forest floor, as it were, where all the negative feelings and hidden impulses lurk in the undergrowth. What we must do is shine a pure light on these shadow creatures—and they will scatter, I promise you. For this we will utilize a very powerful breath that cleans the interior and leaves behind a clear, white space, free from the infestations that create compulsive behavior. I call it the Furnace. It creates the heat necessary to burn away the tangled roots that entrap the unconscious and twist it into harmful knots."

Manhattan was behind us now and we were on the highway. The traffic had become surprisingly, even suspiciously light. I began to wonder if Alan had offered another one of his silent prayers to the potbellied elephant god, Ganesha. I waited expectantly for him to teach me another powerful breathing technique.

Instead he said, "I think this is a good time to tell you more about my father. And me. You will see that addiction is a problem that many of us face at one time or another in our lives."

I listened as Alan enlarged upon the trauma his father had suffered during World War II. On his return to South Africa, he had been unable to settle back into normal life. Loud noises made him jump. His concentration was so poor that he couldn't finish reading the front page of a newspaper. And although he went mechanically to work for Alan's grandfather each day, he accomplished nothing and came home more often than not in a state of drunken disorder.

"I never knew what to expect," Alan said. "Some days he would be angry and aggressive with me, on others sweet-natured and sentimental. I wanted to help, but I was only a child. There was nothing I could do."

Alan's grandfather, a prominent businessman, had been at a loss. He decided to distract Alan's father from his troubles by sending him as his representative on a sales trip to Los Angeles; he was booked into the Ambassador Hotel, which happened to be the same hotel at which a famous yoga guru, Paramahansa Yogananda, was scheduled to give a lecture. Alan's father saw a sign advertising the event and decided to attend. He was so moved by what he heard that afterward, seized by an overwhelming need to know more, he sought out the guru and was permitted to meet with him in private.

"That meeting changed my father's life," Alan said. "He confessed his troubles to Yogananda, who spoke softly and uncritically to him. Although they were meeting for the first time, Yogananda told my father that both he and one of his sons would become yogis. Which is exactly what happened."

"And your father had never done yoga before?"

Alan shook his head.

As soon as Alan's father had returned home to Johannesburg, he left his family and went to India, where he immersed himself in study with Yogananda's brother Bishnu Gosh, another celebrated spiritual teacher. He practiced every day for many months. When he returned to South Africa, he was a new man, purged of his addictions.

But Alan's troubles were not yet over. Although his father had been transformed, Alan remained insecure, vulnerable— and desperately overweight. For some time he had been binge eating and had blown up to 265 pounds. His parents were alarmed. Therapists were engaged. But none was successful. How could they be? Alan did not want to get better. He was confused. He was angry. There were too many painful memories.

"*He* was different," Alan said, "but *I* remained the same. Food was still my only comfort."

"But eventually you made up with him. Right?"

"My father had started to give lessons in yoga. People were talking about how wonderful he was as a teacher. I knew that he could help me, too, but for a long time I stubbornly resisted, out of pride and selfishness. I wanted to hurt him as he had hurt me. One day I could no longer bear the distance between us. I went to him and asked for his help."

Alan's father agreed without hesitation and the next morning came to wake his son at 4:00 A.M. They started practicing together for hours every day. After only three months, Alan had lost a hundred pounds. His anxiety attacks and compulsive behavior soon ceased altogether, and to this day he had never suffered a relapse.

It was not long before Alan's father became such a famous yogi that he was talked of even in India, and their house became a second home to the greatest yogis of the age.

"I remember seeing the portrait in your office of the smiling yogis surrounding you and your father," I said.

"That was how I grew up, tutored by these wise men, who gave freely of their abundant wisdom. Sanskrit became my second language. I didn't have to go to India—the wisdom came to me."

Alan and his father continued to learn and study side by side, eventually creating a new style of yoga that incorporated the great teachings and their own unique ideas. They called it ISHTA, which stands for the Integrated Science of Hatha, Tantra, and Ayurveda.

I looked out of the window as we passed fields of brown and green and yellow, clumps of tall trees in the distance. The countryside seemed so peaceful. More time passed. Alan drove as he lived, freely, but with care and control; at the limit, but not exceeding it.

When we arrived at the conference center, it was approaching dusk. The moon hung like a ghost in the sky, there and not there. We met the organizers and inspected the auditorium, and then Alan spent some time chatting with the guests. He was so easy and frank with them, no one would ever have guessed that he had endured a miserable childhood and conquered a powerful addiction of his own. He inspired me to believe that I could triumph over my own struggles. We still had half an hour before Alan's lecture, and I asked him if he would teach me the Furnace breath.

———————

First, he had me sit down on the floor in a cross-legged position with my hands on my knees, palms facing up, thumbs and first fingers of each hand touching.

Alan asked me to close my eyes and to inhale and exhale gently through my nose a few times. Then he instructed me to exaggerate the movement of my abdomen with each inhalation and exhalation: to really feel my belly push *out* on the inhale, and draw *in* on the exhale, like a bellows fanning a fire. It might feel a bit strange at first, he said, so I should go slowly. When I was comfortable with the rhythm, he wanted me to gradually increase the pace so that the movement became a rapid *in-out, in-out, in-out,* always remembering to push *out* my belly on the inhale, and draw it *in* on the exhale.

Alan watched me work at this for a while. Then he said:

"Try to manage twenty-seven breaths to begin with. While you are breathing, feel a spinning ball of light at the base of your spine slowly expanding and filling your lower body, which will expose and burn away all of your unconscious negative patterns and compulsions, leaving you with a clean, white, empty space inside."

I continued with the breath, even though I wasn't sure that I was getting it.

"Alan, I don't think—"

"That's right, Katrina—*don't* think! Just breathe."

I returned to the rapid *in-out, in-out* breathing pattern.

"Excellent," Alan said, as I approached the last of the twenty-seven breaths. "Now, exhale all the way—keep your eyes closed—and then inhale *completely*. Hold your breath for as long as it feels comfortable, letting your chin drop toward your chest while feeling your belly and pelvic floor drawing in and up (this is called *treta bandha*, or 'triple lock,' because it uses all three *bandhas* at once). Then lift your chin back up as you exhale, sending the light from the base of your spine spiraling up all the way through your body to the crown of the head, releasing it into the air—and with it, all of the unwanted, negative impulses. Sit with your eyes closed, letting your breath return to normal, and just experience the freedom and peace at the core of your being."

When I had finished, I felt euphoric, as if I had left my body and was being pulled toward the moon I had seen a short while ago. After a few minutes I opened my eyes.

"That felt truly amazing."

"When you have more time, aim for four rounds of twenty-seven breaths, for a total of a hundred and eight, and with each round feel that you are penetrating the unconscious more deeply. This technique builds psychic heat, which will burn away all the infestations in your unconscious."

Alan told me to practice for a few weeks; the more I did, the purer and clearer the space inside me would become, and the quicker I would be rid of my burden.

"Like its real-life namesake," he said, "the Furnace needs continual stoking in order to do its job properly. To burn away all vestiges of the old addiction, the internal blaze should be maintained day and night until the job is done."

"Thanks, Alan—thanks so much."

"And one last thing, Katrina."

"Yes?"

"Do not blame yourself for the past."

"I'll try not to."

"Becoming addicted to something is nobody's *fault*. Feeling guilt and shame only allows the negativity to take deeper root inside. And that is the very thing we do not want."

When I got home late that night, there was still no message from Matthew. But I knew I had to be patient. I would try not to panic. There was, however, a message from Ronald. He was still in Hong Kong and wanted to know if I was free the following weekend to visit him in the Hamptons.

Would I see Ronald again? There and then I decided that I wouldn't, however disappointing that might prove to Romilly. Ronald seemed to be the perfect man, but I knew he was not for me. Our lives were too different. He had everything, and I was still trying to find myself. It could never have worked.

What I wanted was a man who was still looking for his own answers. Someone like Matthew. His search for truth was similar to my own. Perhaps that was why I had been attracted to him in the first place. He was the man I wanted, because we were equals and could make our way in life together.

But Matthew was gone. In my impatience to sort out everything in my life, I had driven him away.

Breath Focus 10: FURNACE

Time: 5–20 minutes

Props: none

1. Sit in a comfortable cross-legged position with your spine erect. Let your hands rest on your knees, palms facing upward with the thumbs and first fingers of each hand touching.

2. Close your eyes and take a few slow, deep, natural breaths through your nose. Allow yourself to relax. Inhale and let your belly expand. Exhale and draw your belly in.

3. Now, more forcefully, keeping your mouth closed, inhale fully (press your belly *out* actively) and then exhale by firmly contracting your abdominal muscles to draw your belly *in* toward your spine. Repeat this several times, slowly, and then gradually pick up the pace to find your own rhythm, pumping the abdomen in and out. Work up to twenty-seven full breaths (one breath comprising an inhalation and an exhalation).

4. After twenty-seven breaths, exhale completely, and then inhale fully and hold your breath for as long as is comfortable, dropping your chin toward your chest while feeling your belly and pelvic floor come in and up (*treta bandha*). Draw your awareness to the base of your spine and feel a ball of light—*as powerful as a thousand suns*—burning away any unconscious, harmful impulses and patterns. As you next exhale, let your chin float back up and feel the light travel from the base of your spine out through the crown of your head, releasing these impulses (now rendered inactive) to the Infinite, where they will be dispersed.

5. Repeat for four more rounds, for a total of 108 breaths (in this technique the numbers 27 and 108 are significant because they are multiples of 9, which in yogic philosophy is considered the number of truth).

6. Keeping your eyes closed, let your breath return to normal, and feel the clean, white, empty space inside, now free from all negative infestations. Enjoy the peace and freedom at the core of your being.

(Please note that pregnant women should *not* do this exercise.)

A Note from Katrina

Furnace uses the yogic principle called *tapas*, which is the building of heat to burn out the bad habits and destructive patterns that haunt you. In addition to being an excellent technique for removing obstacles that are buried deep in the unconscious, it is energizing and rejuvenating. Through the rapid succession of sharp, active inhalations and exhalations, the nasal passages are cleansed and purified, the blood is oxygenated, and every cell is re-energized. I find that using this breath makes me feel completely refreshed and full of peace and vitality.

Can this exercise cure an addiction? All I will say is that after practicing it every day for eight months, I felt as if I had finally solved the problem. And it has not been back. Fair warning, though: if you use this breath to help you cure yourself of an addiction, you must give it time to work. Lots of time. A problem that has taken root over many years cannot be eradicated in an hour. You may want to give up, as we all sometimes do with difficult tasks—but be patient, keep going, and you will surely get worthwhile results.

More than any one exercise, however, curing yourself of an addiction comes down to establishing a real sense of self: the more you feel you are the person you were meant to be, the less you need to look elsewhere for comfort. If you have been faithfully following the exercises in this book, I am confident that your new, true self is now becoming more apparent with every day.

A lot of women suffer from addictions of one sort or another. It is nothing to be ashamed of. The pressures on us throughout our lives are enormous, first from our own families, and then from the families we create, or hope to create. Every day, someone is telling us what to do. *Try this. Do that. Take more. Give more.* These multiple and insistent messages serve only to confuse and distract us from our paths.

Use the Furnace, and, over time, you will burn away the impulses that threaten to become, or have already been transformed into, an addiction. Remember that the true you is always there inside, waiting quietly to be rediscovered.

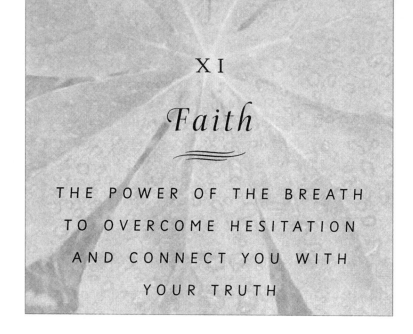

XI

Faith

THE POWER OF THE BREATH
TO OVERCOME HESITATION
AND CONNECT YOU WITH
YOUR TRUTH

Somehow it seemed absolutely right that Halloween was to be the night of my big test. I was hoping for a night of magic, a night when the spirits would make contact with the physical world—or at least with me, because I would be demonstrating yoga poses onstage with Alan at the closing event of one of North America's biggest annual yoga conferences, which was being held this year in Miami.

This was a different kind of Halloween from the one I had grown up with: no damp weather, no falling leaves, no sepia sky. Just sun, sun, sun—and palm trees. Blue sea and blue sky joined together in a hazy blur at the horizon.

I was thrilled that Alan had asked me to be his demonstrator at this important event. And nervous. There were many more accomplished yoga students at the studio, but Alan said he wanted me. I would be appearing in front of a live audience—hundreds of serious yoga students and teachers had paid to stay at this luxury hotel and attend Alan's demonstration in the conference center's massive auditorium.

The last time I had been on a stage, I was five and wearing traditional Ukrainian dress for the Christmas school pageant. All I had to do was look cute and say the Ukrainian word for Christmas at the right moment. But my mind went blank, and for a whole minute I stood there, my face getting redder and redder. The audience was snickering. Then the teacher, offstage, prompted me in a loud whisper. What if I froze up again? I'd be finished. Even worse, Alan's reputation would be. I couldn't bear that.

———

The conference was spread out over four days and three nights. I had one small bag, and Alan had brought two huge suitcases, a carry-on, and a backpack.

"I know, I know," he said, when I goggled at his luggage. "I take everything in the house. But I need to be ready—I never know where the Universe will send me!"

There were many different events going on during the long weekend of the conference, with teachers and gurus from all over the United States. Although Alan was one of the main attractions, there were several younger rising stars of yoga who were also getting a lot of publicity. It turned out that two of the biggest new names were Alan's former students. I asked him how he felt about that. He was delighted for them.

On the second morning, something unexpected happened.

Alan and I had just finished a workshop, and he had gone to his room to freshen up before lunch. I noticed a guy hanging around, and when he saw Alan enter the elevator he approached me.

"Hey."

"Hi," I said. "Can I help you?" He looked sort of familiar.

"My name is Byron Makepeace. And you're Katrina, right?"

I knew the name, of course: he was a successful yogi, known for an intense physical style of yoga. With his surfer good looks and cool, he had attracted a celebrity clientele and was especially popular with music and film folk. His hair was different from the picture I had seen of him in *Yoga Journal*. There it had been long; now it was short, almost cropped. Several of his followers were standing a short distance away. They were all young and good-looking.

"Mr. Make—"

"Byron. Please." He moved closer. "I've been watching you."

"Why?"

"Why?" He let out a short laugh, then reined it back in just as quickly. He had cold eyes, like some glinting stone you might find lying at the bottom of the sea. "I'm opening a studio in Manhattan. I want you to come and work for me."

"Thanks, Byron, but I work for Alan."

"I understand. You're loyal." He turned the thick leather band that encircled his wrist. "Loyalty? It's a princely quality. I do admire it. What's he paying you?"

"That's not—"

"I need an assistant and I want you. I'll pay a hundred thousand dollars a year. To start."

"Byr—"

"And benefits. Health. Pension. We look after our people at Locus Yoga."

He smiled at me. Although you could say he was attractive, there was something about his wide grin that suggested hollowness. Perhaps because it was Halloween, his face was beginning to remind me of a jack-o'-lantern.

"Locus Yoga," I said. "That's Latin, isn't it? Not Sanskrit."

"Well spotted," Byron said. "*Locus* is Latin for 'place,' and Locus Yoga is the place to go. But, between you, me, and the Great Buddha—*shanti, shanti*—there is also the suggestion of the word *locust*. As in we are going to cover the world. Like it?"

"Clever," I said. "Very clever." *But didn't locusts eat everything in their path?*

"And you'd be *clever* to join me, Katrina. Once I see someone I like, I don't often let go. Don't give me your answer now. Think on it, and then say yes. Come to my workshop tonight: Playing the Divine Game of Life to Win. It's very spiritual. Entry is a hundred and fifty dollars. But I'll leave your name at the door."

He turned with the grace of a ballet dancer and marched off with his group, leaving a trace of sandalwood in the air.

A hundred thousand dollars a year. A princely sum, Byron might call it. I wouldn't have to worry about whether I could stay in New York. Or where to live. I could live where I liked and be independent. But right now was not the time to make a decision.

I set aside Byron's offer and concentrated on the days ahead.

———

In the late afternoon before Alan's final keynote event, he and I walked down to the main shopping area together for an early supper at a Mexican restaurant.

"Charlie is very enthusiastic about your becoming a teacher," Alan said while we ate. "She has mentioned it to me several times. Are you considering it?"

"I'd love to teach."

"That's why I recommend that you take the teacher-training course. There's one starting in January."

I went on eating.

"Why do you hesitate?" he said.

"I don't know. I just don't feel ready yet."

"How long have we been working together?"

"Nearly a year."

"You are a very different person from the Katrina I met a year ago."

"Thanks to you."

"And you are ready for the next stage of self-discovery," he said.

"I don't feel ready," I said. "Not really."

"It's time," he said. "Time to take the next step for yourself."

I nodded. But I didn't want to take the next step for myself. In spite of everything I had learned, I still felt as if I needed Alan's guidance to make the right decisions.

I thought then of a film I had seen many years before, *The Red Balloon*, and how the balloon floats away over the rooftops of Paris. All of a sudden I felt certain that Alan was about to let go of me, too, like the red balloon.

We went back to the hotel and retired to our rooms to prepare for the evening. I tried to nap but couldn't—I was too excited. And now, with just over an hour to go before the show, I was becoming more and more agitated.

My room was on the twentieth floor of one of the dozen

luxury hotels that line the beachfront of Bal Harbour, the upscale resort "village" north of the city of Miami. The whole place had been built from scratch with one intention: to part you from your money. There were luxury spas and luxury suites and luxury shops. I had already done the main street, Collins Avenue, where I stared into the windows of Bulgari and Cartier, Prada and Tiffany. Byron Makepeace's offer came back to me. A hundred thousand dollars. With such a salary, I could buy some awfully nice things.

I realized with a jolt that, if I accepted his offer, not only would I solve one of my permanently nagging worries—money—but I'd impress my father.

"And that's not all, Dad," I imagined myself saying. "I get health benefits and I can join the company pension plan."

"And you say this is all from doing handstands?"

"Yoga, Dad."

"Wait till I tell my golfing buddies. A hundred thousand dollars for doing handstands! They'll laugh their shoelaces off. The world's gone crazy!"

"Perhaps it has, Dad," I would say. "But I won't need to borrow any money from you now to get a mortgage."

He'd have to revise his previous reservations about my "lifestyle."

Charlie would not have liked this kind of talk. Getting rich from yoga was very unspiritual in her eyes. Then again, Alan had no qualms about living well; money was quite acceptable to a disciple of Tantra. He charged some of his wealthy clients top dollar, although what he took from them he gave back tenfold in time and attention to people like me. That was how to live with yourself when you earned a lot of money, I thought. You had to give back, and it wasn't enough just to donate money; no, the only real way to give back was with your *time*.

———

A week before the conference, Lisa and I had taken a walk from the south entrance of Central Park all the way to the northern perimeter. It had been a misty, dusky day, quite lovely. The trees were in full fall splendor. For me, this is the most romantic season.

I was glad to have Lisa as my friend; we could talk freely about art and writing and family. Although I was fond of Romilly, she only wanted to discuss the next thing to do on her "life list." And our last conversation had not been pleasant: she had been disappointed with me when I told her that I would not be seeing Ronald Hass again. She even sounded rather angry. "I thought we understood each other," she said. "If you want to make it in New York, you don't look the other way when opportunity calls." And she hadn't spoken to me since. I decided not to call her with any sort of apology. I used to chase after people I liked who were upset with me and try to explain myself, but I was stronger now. If Romilly had dropped me, then it was her loss.

I still hadn't heard from Matthew. In the past month, I had gone through a range of emotions: anger at myself for giving him an ultimatum, and then at him for not being in touch; guilt over my date with Ronald; sadness that our relationship might be over; anxiety about how I would make it on my own; and then, finally, resignation—I'd put him on the back burner and turned it down to low heat. What will happen, will happen, Alan said. But I thought I'd call home and check my messages anyway. It would take my mind off tonight's rapidly approaching panic attack.

Nothing from Matthew. But there was a message.

"Hello, dear, it's Mom. Thought I'd catch you this time, but I've probably miscalculated the time difference. I just got back from the mechanic's, where I had the oil replaced and winter tires put on the car, and now I am carving a pumpkin and roasting the seeds to go on a feta salad that I am having for dinner. Remember that year when I made the princess costume for you and you were on the local news? Those were special times. I love you. Happy Halloween!"

I put down the phone and suddenly felt like crying. I remembered how she used to cut my sandwiches into heart shapes and write me little notes on the napkins she put in my lunch box. All the things she had done for me while I was growing up. I wouldn't be here without all her love and care. Even though my last trip home had been difficult, I had finally come to accept our relationship as it was, and that had brought me peace of mind. There were some things we would never agree on, but they wouldn't stand in the way of my love for her.

Feeling I could use some reassurance, I called her, but she wasn't in. I left a message.

"It's Katrina. I'm in Miami with Alan at a big yoga conference. We're going onstage soon. I just wanted to thank you for everything you've done for me. I'm not sure if I've ever told you that before. I love you lots, Mom. Bye for now."

I felt so much better after doing that.

The sun was going down. I checked my watch. Time to get ready. My heart was beating too fast. I sat cross-legged on the floor and did some breathing exercises. Then I undressed and got into the shower. The water was soothing, but I still felt jumpy. Why couldn't I relax? Under the pulsing showerhead, I thought of all the things that could go wrong at the big event:

1. I pull a muscle in my leg doing the Warrior pose and have to perform for the rest of the evening in a crouch.
2. I walk too close to the front of the stage and fall off.
3. I do the wrong pose for Alan and this throws me and the audience starts booing and I mess up all the others.
4. Because of this, Byron Makepeace lowers his offer to $40,000.

This was ridiculous! I got out of the shower and dried myself. It was still too early to meet with Alan.

I went up to the window and pressed my nose to the glass. There was a sheer, unobstructed drop to the ground. Nothing at the bottom but a thin strip of road, then sand dotted with palms, and then the vast emptiness of the sea. Suddenly I felt dizzy and had to look up. Miami was just starting its daily ritual at sundown: orange and yellow bursts with streaks of pink. Very striking. But all I could think about was that I would be standing in front of hundreds of people in less than half an hour.

I had never really admitted it to myself, but I was terrified of being onstage. That was why I hadn't felt ready to be a teacher. And that was why I just had to grit my teeth and go out there and kick ass. But my damn hands were shaking.

Okay, whatever. Time to go. I picked up my jacket, my mat, and my gym bag, and closed the door behind me. No turning back now. My legs seemed to weigh five hundred pounds apiece. Every step down the long corridor to Alan's room was a huge effort. At last I got there. I was almost gasping for air. I knocked.

"Perfect timing," he said. "I just finished my meditation."

That was what I should have been doing. If my mind had only let me.

We took the elevator down to the third floor and joined the walkway leading to the conference center.

"You're very quiet," Alan said. "Everything okay?"

"Al, I'm scared sick. I thought everything was under control, but I realize that I have this phobia about appearing in public. I've never done it before, not like this. And there are going to be so many people!"

"Relax," he said, "everything will be just fine." He patted me on the shoulder. But it wasn't. And it was getting worse. I thought I might have to run off at any moment. It would be very hard to find me in the basement of a hotel: there are always endless corridors and hallways and laundry rooms and tangles of pipes. I could hide out in the shadows until it was all over.

We arrived at the hall, and the manager gave us a quick tour. It was a huge cavern, a train station of a hall. You could hold a Super Bowl in there. Then the stage manager came over and had a brief talk with us. Any special lighting requirements? No, Alan said. Yes, I said. Can we have them all off? With horror I saw that the audience was already filing in.

We were shown to a dressing room, and Alan suggested we do some breathing exercises together. He spoke softly and his voice calmed me. My breathing became slower and steadier. For five minutes I felt better and better. Then there was a knock on the door.

"Folks, we're ready for you to begin, whenever you are."

"Thank you," Alan said. "We'll be out in two minutes."

Alan looked at me and frowned. "Still anxious?"

"Terrified. I don't think I can go out there."

"Everything will be fine," he said. "Just relax, sit up tall, and close your eyes."

I sat like that for a minute.

Then I felt Alan tap on the center of my forehead three times.

Straightaway I felt a powerful energy radiating through my head and then diffusing throughout my body, followed by a gentle pulsation moving up from the base of my spine to the crown of my head.

My mind grew quieter, calmer, then completely calm, and then . . . empty.

I began to feel waves of peaceful stillness washing over me (like warm shivers running up and down my spine).

Immediately, all my fear vanished.

I fell into a state between dreaming and waking: comfortable, secure, blissful.

Although Alan had never done this for me before, I knew what was happening, even with my eyes closed. At that moment his hand was positioned several inches above my head, drawing energy up from the base of my spine to my crown. It was an ancient yogic technique called *shaktipat,* the transfer of spiritual energy from Master Yogi to student, which is said to give the student an experience of the Divine. Alan was one of only a handful of Western masters who had been initiated into the practice, and he had promised to share it with me one day, when I really needed it. I'd never needed it more.

I must have been in a dream state for a few minutes, although it felt like seconds.

"How do you feel now?" he asked.

I opened my eyes. "Wonderful."

"Then let's show our audience the wonder of yoga."

We walked down the corridor that led to the auditorium, climbed the steps—and were suddenly onstage. The lights were raised and Alan walked toward the front of the stage, with me following behind. I no longer felt afraid. I was ready.

"Namaste!" Alan announced to the crowd through the mini-microphone that the stage manager had pinned to his shirt. The audience immediately quieted down.

Alan sat cross-legged and the audience followed. Then he put his hands together in front of his heart and bowed his head.

"Welcome, everyone," he said. "Today we will start off with a meditation, and then *asana*, for which the poses will be demonstrated by my assistant, Katrina."

An hour into the show, it was going very well. My demonstration had, as far as I could tell, been almost perfect. I glided from one pose to the next without thinking or hesitating; I was glad I had spent so much time preparing my routine. Far from being afraid now, I began to relish the presence of the audience and feed off their energy. It was amazing to look out of the corner of my eye and see all those people copying what I was doing.

I was onstage, in front of an audience, performing. I had done it, with Alan's help. All I had to do now was finish without falling on my butt.

Two hours later we were back in the dressing room. I had sweated clean through my outfit. I probably looked awful, but I felt great. Alan was exhausted but exhilarated. The event had been an outstanding success. It was an amazing feeling.

"Thank you, Katrina. You did great work out there."

"Thanks to you," I said.

"Come on," Alan said, "let's get our stuff and go upstairs."

There was a crowd of people outside the conference center waiting for Alan to emerge. He spent a few minutes chatting and signing programs. I hung back, but several people noticed me and came over to say how much they had enjoyed my performance. Then I noticed Byron Makepeace. While Alan was still occupied, he approached me.

"Now are you ready to come and work for me?" he said, giving me his jack-o'-lantern grin.

"No," I said. "I'm turning down your offer. Thanks very much."

Byron's grin fell off his face.

"You'd turn down a hundred thousand dollars? How stupid can you be?"

"Stupid or not," I said, "I'm sticking with Alan."

Byron shook his head and walked off without another word.

"So he was trying to steal you away, was he?" Alan asked, coming up beside me.

"He did offer me a lot of money," I replied. "But he's not my style. I could never have worked for him."

"I understand that he's opening a studio in Manhattan," Alan said. "And he's looking for good people."

"I'm sure he'll find plenty of willing takers. I did think about it—I'd have been a fool not to. Having that kind of money would settle a lot of my anxieties about the future. But I just know that working for him would raise a whole host of other problems. Besides which, I believe in loyalty."

Alan smiled and nodded, but did not respond.

When we had arrived at our floor, I expected us to say our goodnights, but Alan asked me to leave everything in my room except my mat and come with him to the roof garden.

"It's a beautiful night," he said. "Perfect conditions for the last breath I want to teach you. Your year of learning is almost complete."

I dropped my bag in my room and joined Alan once more at the elevator. We rose another five floors to the roof garden, which was lit discreetly around the perimeter of a swimming pool whose surface rippled gently in the breeze, sometimes giving off flashes of silvery light when it reflected the moon. We were alone. There was a faint murmur of people and cars far below.

As a university student, I had worked at the Calgary Planetarium and been fascinated by the moon's surface. That night it was so close I could count the craters. There was something sad about its old, pockmarked face. The sky was a shifting blue-black, and the stars were countless sparkling pinholes. I could make out the Big Dipper. The vastness of the sky did not feel at all daunting. I was still high from the show.

"Let's lay out our mats here," Alan said.

We sat cross-legged, facing each other. Alan looked up at the stars for a moment, then turned his attention to me.

"Very beautiful," he said.

I nodded.

"I am proud of you, Katrina. You have made remarkable progress during our year together."

"Thank you." I could feel myself becoming more emotional. *Don't be silly.*

"There comes a time when knowledge must be put into practice. Now is your time. You are ready."

"For what?" I said.

"To move to the next stage of your personal development. To become the person you were always meant to be."

"But I'm still not sure who I'm meant to be."

"You are. Inside. Everything we have been doing together since that first day you took my class has been leading to this moment. That's why I wanted us to see the sky tonight. In ancient times, man was the center of the Universe and everything revolved around him. Everything was in harmony. Over the millennia we have lost faith in that harmony, in the certainty that each one of us is the center. It has been my role to restore you to your center—to help you see that you are part of the Universe and the Universe is part of you. That everything outside is also inside. That you have everything you need. You always did."

"I believe that now, Alan. But what happens next?"

"What happens next, happens without me."

"Without you—?"

"I am going to show you a breath that will connect you with everything in the Universe. It will give you the one remaining element you still lack—faith in yourself."

———

The breath was called Horizon. Alan explained that as the horizon is the line that joins earth and sky, so the Horizon breath would take me to the point at which matter and spirit unite—the Infinite.

"To experience the Infinite," he said, "we make use of the most powerful weapon known to yogis—the sound of *Om*."

Alan explained that *Om* is what is known in yoga as a *mantra,* which is a sound vibration that is used to alter one's consciousness. *Mantra* comes from the Sanskrit words *manas* (mind) and *tra* (liberation): it is a tool that is used to liberate the mind. The sound of *Om* is considered a seed sound that contains all knowledge, all potential, all inspiration— everything. It is the vibrating, pulsing energy of the Universe itself and drives away all hesitation and uncertainty.

Om is composed of four parts: the sounds *ahh*, *ohh*, *mmm*, and silence.

Ahh is the rawest sound that you can make: it starts at the back of the throat and vibrates at the base of the spine.

Ohh is formed at the roof of the mouth and vibrates in the heart center.

Mmm uses the gums and lips to move the energetic vibration to the crown of the head. When the sound dies away, you sit absorbed in the silence.

"Then you are at the Horizon point—where matter and spirit meet," Alan said.

"What do I do?"

"First of all, just experiment with the sounds. Try the *ahh*, and notice how it vibrates near the base of your spine (you can even place a hand on your lower belly to help you). Then practice the *ohh* and feel how the vibration moves up to your heart. Finally, feel the *mmm* as it vibrates through your skull. And then just sit in the silence."

I experimented. I grasped what Alan meant almost immediately.

"Now close your eyes, place your thumbs at the entrances to your ears, spread your fingers, and let the tips rest lightly on the top of your skull. Take a deep breath in, and when you exhale, move through the *ahh* and *ohh* sounds. When you come to the *mmm*, plug your ears, and at the same time draw your fingers gently apart (the action is akin to opening your skull). This technique increases the resonance (a sort of stereo effect), and really helps to enhance the wholeness of the vibration, which will continue to be felt afterward."

I tried it out.

"Repeat the breath nine times. At the end of each breath, feel the vibration at the center of your brain radiating outward, as if the crown of your head were opening up. Do you feel it? Imagine actually being drawn toward the horizon. Listen to the *mmm* until you run out of breath, and then rest quietly, bathing in the silence of the sound beyond sound. That is the final stage and the purest form of *Om*."

I did as Alan suggested, and then paused after each breath to absorb the silence. It was astonishing. I could still feel a humming sound in my ears. It was as though all of the pulsations and all of the vibrations in the Universe were inside me, moving through me and around me.

I just sort of let go. The vastness of the night sky, the stars, the wind, the sounds far below—everything seemed to enter me and lift me up, until I felt as if I were full of energy and life and had begun to float upward on the air currents. Up and up I went, higher and higher, until I was far above the roof garden. Down below I could see Alan getting smaller and smaller. I was disappearing into the night sky to be lost among the stars.

I was the red balloon—and I was free.

For what seemed like hours, I floated in the heavens, all the while sure that I could not fall. What had I been afraid of, all this time? The future? But how could I be afraid of the unknown, when it seemed to me now that the future was everything I wanted it to be? All this time my fears had been about silly, stupid things—and now that I believed in myself those fears had simply gone. The Universe would protect and guide me.

Gradually I felt myself floating back down to my position on the roof. I just seemed to settle back into myself again. Afterward I felt absolutely at peace. Everything was as it should be.

The night wind caressed my face. I opened my eyes. *For the first time in my life I wasn't afraid.*

Without anticipating it, I experienced a wave of immense gratitude to Alan, his teachers, and all of the people who had been a part of my journey so far. I inwardly gave thanks to my parents for giving birth to me, and also for each and every experience—good and bad—that had brought me to this present moment.

"Do you feel ready now?" Alan asked.

"Yes," I said. "I'm going to become a yoga teacher."

Later in my room, after a long hot shower, I was lying happily on the bed, slowly falling to sleep. My cell rang. I flipped it open. The first thing I heard was . . . sobbing? I sat up.

"Who's there?"

A very quiet voice said: "Katrina? It's Romilly. I—I'm sorry to call so late."

"Romilly?" This didn't sound like her. I sat up. "What is it? What's wrong?"

She sniffed. "The bastard just kicked me out of his bed and sent me home. I'm sick of men. Sick of them. They're all the same."

There was a noise. I thought she must have dropped the phone. Then she said, "Sorry. Are you still there?"

"Of course."

"I can't talk to the other girls about this. They'd think I was being weak. But I'm not. I tried so hard to make him love me."

"Who, Romilly?"

There was a silence.

"It's okay if you don't want to talk about it."

"I do, I do," she said. "But promise not to be angry with me."

"Why? What are you talking about?"

"For Ronald."

"Ronald . . . Hass? What's he got to do with it?"

"That's who just sent me home."

"But you told me—"

"I know. I'm sorry. I lied. I was so in love with him, can you understand? So in love that I was willing to do anything that might make him grateful to me. I was even willing to share him with you, if that's what he wanted. But you didn't go for it. Now he's mad at me."

So Romilly had set me up. I was about to say something unpleasant and hang up, but that wouldn't have helped. And, to tell the truth, I was relieved. Now I wouldn't have to wonder what might have happened with Ronald. My initial flash of anger was quickly replaced with pity. I wasn't the one who was suffering. Romilly had called me for help. I couldn't let her down.

We talked. She had been dating Ronald for about a year, was crazy about him. He kept promising an engagement but always put her off when she mentioned it. And she just got in deeper and deeper. He would call her over in the middle of the night. Sometimes he would make a date and then stand her up. It just made her want him more. He was the ultimate New York catch. Money. Looks. And a cold heart. And then he had asked her to set him up with me.

"Will you ever forgive me?" she said.

"I already have."

"I'm going to change," she said. "I've had enough of this way of living. Will you help me? I trust you."

"You must be going through hell, Rom. But don't forget

that whatever Ronald has done to you, he can't take away what's inside. You're still the same gorgeous, smart woman. And I'm here for you whenever you need me."

"Thank you, Katrina. Thank you so much for understanding."

We promised to get together when I returned to the city.

The next day Alan and I flew back to New York. It was a bumpy flight, and normally I would have been gripping the armrests, but somehow it didn't affect me the way it usually did. Something had changed.

And when I arrived home in the early evening, I found something else had changed.

Matthew was back.

Breath Focus 11: HORIZON

Time: 5–20 minutes

Props: none

1. Find a quiet place away from distraction and sit cross-legged.

2. Close your eyes and tune in to your breath.

3. Place your thumbs in the entrances to your ears and spread your fingers so that the tips rest on the top of your head.

4. Breathe in deeply.

5. As you breathe out, make the sound of *ahh*: feel it vibrating at the base of your spine. Then *ohh*: feel the vibration moving up to your heart. Finally, plug your ears and draw your fingers slightly apart as you make the sound of *mmm*, feeling the vibration in your skull. This is the sound of *Om*. (The *ahh*, *ohh*, and *mmm* should be three equal parts of one exhalation, held for as long as is comfortable for you.)

6. At the end of the exhalation, let yourself sit for a few moments in the silence, feeling the oneness at the core of your being.

7. Repeat nine times.

A Note from Katrina

Because this breath is audible (like Ocean Breath), it may require a few test runs before you become accustomed to it.

Once you have internalized the sensation of *Om*, it is not even necessary to make the sound. You can simply focus silently on the *ahh, ohh, mmm* moving up the spine. And then concentrate on the silence—the sound behind the sound.

Om teaches you that everything is as it should be. Over time, the sound will become a part of you that you can summon at will to tune in to the Universe. Whenever you feel the onset of doubts about your future or yourself, use this breath. You will more than likely find, as I did, that as the months pass you are less and less afraid of making the decisions that will enable you to become the person you have always wanted to be.

Using the Horizon breath allows us to return again and again to the point at which spirit and matter meet. We can tap into the infinite spiritual space beyond, and feel peace and a union with all things. Once we are connected to the Universe, we know we are on the right path.

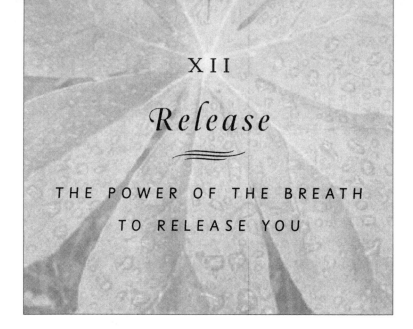

XII

Release

THE POWER OF THE BREATH

TO RELEASE YOU

I entered the room and put down my bag. Matthew was working at his laptop. He turned around and smiled.

"Hi," he said. "You're back."

"So are you, it seems. For good?"

"I decided that I do want to be here in New York."

He got up and walked toward me. "With you."

We hugged. At first I felt a bit awkward. After weeks of imagining our reconciliation and then almost giving up hope, it was strange to embrace as though we had never been apart. But it didn't take long for me to realize that I really was overjoyed to see Matthew again.

We sat down, and he told me how he had taken a couple of

Mark's classes at Penn but found that his mind just wasn't on the work. One night the two of them had talked it through at a local pub and Mark had persuaded Matthew to try again with me.

"Not that it took much persuading," Matthew said. I was grateful that Mark was a writer; writers always seem to be sympathetic people.

Then Matthew said, "I've got a little surprise."

He went to the kitchen and pulled out a bottle of Mumm's champagne.

"Shall we?"

I couldn't help smiling.

As we drank, I told him all about the conference in Miami and how I had made the decision to become a yoga teacher. It wasn't too long before the bottle was empty and we were light-headed, so we went out for dinner to the sushi place around the corner, and later I slept better than I had the whole time Matthew was away.

The next morning it really felt as if we were starting afresh. I apologized again for giving him an ultimatum, and he apologized again for running off.

Now that he was talking to me, Matthew seemed keen for us to spend time together. He had to leave for a meeting with his MFA adviser at school, but we made a date for lunch at our favorite organic restaurant—we were both desperate for steamed vegetables and rice, neither one of us having eaten very healthily recently. I thought about my pizza episode and decided to say nothing. It seemed so incredible now, as if it had never happened. Who was that person? It wasn't me—it was some crazy lady I wouldn't be bumping into again, I hoped.

Outside the sky was a crisp and sunlit blue—one of those

rare fall days in New York that are like jewels you want to keep locked up in a box for the rest of the year, to enjoy them again at your leisure. I decided to go for a long walk before our lunch.

I was just about to leave the apartment when the phone rang. My father was on the line. It was National Beaver Day or something in Canada and he wanted to wish me a happy one.

"Thanks, Dad," I said. "And how are you?"

"Oh, not so bad. My golf's been off. I think I'll give it up, it's too much effort."

It was not the first time my dad had made such a statement; actually, it happened every year. And every year he went back for more, playing an average of three to four games a week.

"Come on, Dad, you can't give up your favorite game. You're so good at it."

"Maybe it's time for a change. I've been watching a lot of Oprah recently."

He had recently retired and was well acquainted with daytime TV, which was now just the warm-up to his already packed evening viewing schedule of sports, news, and movies. Golfing was his last link with the outside world, and I dreaded to think what would happen if he stopped.

"Dad, you shouldn't be sitting in the house all afternoon. It's not healthy."

"What else am I going to do? That Dr. Phil reminds me of Bryan Goberman from my old office. Same mustache. Of course, Bryan was found guilty of misappropriating company funds, so there the similarity ends."

I waited for Dad to say more, but he must have been waiting for me, so I said, "What kind of change are you talking about?"

But he said, "Do you remember when I taught you how to ride a bike?"

"Of course I do, Dad."

"What a day that was. Off you went, your little legs pedaling like—what's that damn word?"

"Pistons?"

"That's it. Down the hill you went with me running after you. We had some good times together. I know we had some rough times, too—but there were good times, weren't there?"

"Plenty," I said. "You taught me how to ski, remember? And play golf."

"And we used to play catch in the backyard when I came home from work." He sighed. "All those years ago."

Silence.

"And the zoo, Dad, remember? You loved to take me to the zoo."

"Didn't I say that with all your energy and pranks you belonged in the monkey house?"

"Yes, Dad, you did. And what about our trip to Russia and the Ukraine to visit your relatives?"

"Oh, yes!"

On a couple of occasions we both drank way too much vodka. Which was a real blast for a sixteen-year-old.

"Have I been a good father to you?"

"Of course, Dad."

"I'm glad. Sometimes I think—"

"Dad, I'm going to stay in New York and become a yoga teacher."

"What? You don't—?"

"I do. I've made up my mind. I'm sorry if that's disappointing to you. I don't want to go back into the corporate world."

I realized I was holding my breath. *Breathe,* I told myself. One deep breath, two, three. I braced myself for the inevitable criticism and lecture.

"Well, well, well."

Here we go. He's building up some pressure. Getting ready to spout. Well, I'm not backing down this time. Not this time, Dad.

"You're angry," I said.

"Angry? Not at all—I'm proud of you. You're finally working out what it is you want to do. That's wonderful. What is it that fella on the TV who wrote that book says—'Follow your bliss'?"

I couldn't believe it. "So you don't mind?" *And can I have it in writing, please?*

"Mind? Not a bit. Long as you come back home for Christmas. I'm going to cook a meal for you—and that man you live with."

"Matthew."

"Well, I won't cook it, exactly—you will. When are you people getting married, then?"

"Don't hold your breath, Dad."

"I'm going to have a good long talk with him when he gets here."

I was laughing as we said our goodbyes. With relief, no doubt. His approval was just so important to me. He didn't think I was wasting my time! I felt like sending flowers to Oprah and Dr. Phil. Dad really *was* changing. Maybe during my visit at Christmas I could get him started on Alan's breathing exercises . . .

I left the apartment and wandered through the noisy, dirty, chaotic city streets I had come to love. Is there a better feeling than having a whole morning free with nothing to worry about and nothing to do but roam around looking at things? Free time. It was a greater luxury than the newest Prada bag. I spent the next couple of hours just enjoying the feeling of being alone but not lonely. I was so content, I did not even have the desire to buy anything or be anyone but myself.

I really was on my way. Heading in the right direction, too, this time. I was going to be a yoga teacher. But try as I might not to, I worried what people back home would think of me when I told them. Even after that amazing session on the rooftop of the Miami hotel, and what it had taught me, I was still sensitive to others' opinions. To most of my old friends, yoga was just something you did in your spare time (if at all), not a career. They'd probably think I was a slacker. Did that matter? It still did, somehow. My indoctrination—the idea of what constitutes success and failure in life—was so complete that I knew I still had a struggle ahead. It wasn't a matter of convincing them—I had to convince myself.

And then there was Matthew: what would happen if he couldn't make it as a writer? Over the past year he'd regained some of the money he had lost in the markets, but could he survive without having to go back to work in some cubicle and give up on his dream? And if he failed, how would that affect me?

And what about the family I wanted to start?

There were real obstacles ahead of us. And even with all of Alan's teachings (and prayers to Ganesha, the Great Remover), these obstacles would not miraculously disappear.

The beauty of the morning began to fade the more I thought about what lay ahead. Having come this far in changing my life, would I have to do an about-face on the brink of success and back down? The traffic noise suddenly changed from symphony to cacophony. Why couldn't people walk faster? They hogged the center of the pavement and had conversations with their friends ten feet away! And look at that guy spitting on the street. I hated spitters. But they were always the type who would knife you if you so much as gave them a look.

God, what was happening to me? I'd already lost the magic I had earlier. I needed reassurance. I needed to talk with Matthew. I made my way to the restaurant and sat down opposite him. He closed the book he had been reading.

"What's wrong?" he said. "You've got that look."

"I'm anxious."

I told him how everything still seemed so impossible. How would we ever have enough money to buy an apartment, have a child, and live without being stressed out all the time? Matthew took my hands in his and told me that the important thing was to stick together, and if we could do that, things would surely work out for us.

"Do you really believe that?" I said.

"I do. We'll have to make a few sacrifices, but we'll pull through."

"Okay. But I do definitely want a baby."

Matthew burst out laughing. "You don't stop, do you?" he said.

I smiled. *No. Not until I get what I want. Especially when I know it's what you really want, too.*

Our lunch had arrived. We both set to work on downtown's best bowl of steamed vegetables and rice.

"One more thing," Matthew said. "If you want us to stay together and be happy, you have to be prepared for uncertainty. The way we will live—writing, teaching yoga—means that there will be little security at first. But I believe that real security comes from being happy in your work. And being good at it, of course. If we aim for that, we'll make it. You'll see."

I nodded. What will happen, will happen. Why was I still trying to control the future?

One thing was certain: having come this far together, I didn't want to give up on him now. I could make all the changes I wanted to *my* life, but I shouldn't try to change Matthew. Besides, he was too strong for that. It was up to me to take him for who he was, not for what I might want him to be. If I loved him—really loved him, and wasn't just pretending—then he could be the person he was and I would be happy with that. And I was, wasn't I?

I thought about all those Hollywood romantic comedies that I loved so much. After overcoming the usual misunderstandings and setbacks, the boy and girl always end up in each other's arms, and as they kiss passionately, the film ends and the audience goes away thinking everything is bluebirds and daisies and sunshine ever after.

But it wasn't. Hollywood had it all wrong. That was just the end of Stage One. The next stage was the hard part. That was when you found out if you really had chosen the right person.

———

A month passed. The day before Thanksgiving I had an appointment at the studio to record some more of Alan's teachings, after which he had invited me to join in the group meditation he was organizing for all the teachers and trainees, even though my training didn't begin officially until the new year. Then there was a drinks party for Charlie, who was leaving to go traveling in India.

Already the Christmas lights and decorations were looped around the lampposts and hanging still unlit above the streets. I walked through Union Square, where they were just putting up the outdoor Christmas market. That always gave me a warm feeling. I loved to wander in the late afternoon among the stalls with their scented candles and stuffed pillows and Christmas novelties, as much for the sights and smells as for the proximity to other folk eagerly anticipating the start of the holiday season. It was kitschy, and I lapped it up.

I arrived at the studio just as the three o'clock pregnancy yoga class was about to start. Clustered around the reception desk was a group of chattering women. They all looked radiant, and I felt such a bond with them that I knew one day I would have my own child. And there and then I had an overwhelming feeling that Matthew would be the father.

A familiar head appeared from behind the office door.

"Come in, future teacher!" Alan waved me into his private room.

For the next hour we drank tea and discussed the Eight Limbs of Yoga, as described in the Yoga Sutras, while I recorded and made notes. When Alan had finished talking, he invited Matthew and me to join him and his family at their annual dinner, which was to be held this year at a restaurant in SoHo.

I thanked him but said that Matthew and I planned to spend this Thanksgiving together, alone.

"I have so much to be grateful for," I said. "Beginning with everything you've given me this past year. I feel as if I have made great progress toward finding my truth."

"And you will continue to make progress, I am sure," Alan said. "Next year you will train to be a teacher. I have no doubt that you will be a very good one."

"You sound so confident," I said. "I wish I could be. I still need reassurance that everything will work out. The future looks so uncertain."

"Your future is more certain than you know," Alan said. "I will show you why. Before the meditation starts, I have one more lesson to give you."

What—only one more? Surely there were hundreds more.

"The lesson is this: you must let go."

Immediately the picture of the red balloon appeared again in my head.

"I think I already did let go, Al." I told him about the red balloon.

"Ah, but you saw only half the picture. Close your eyes for a moment. Imagine you are the red balloon again. You are floating over the rooftops. You are looking ahead and away into the distance."

I closed my eyes. "Okay."

"Now look down."

I did—and saw that although I seemed to be floating freely, I wasn't.

I opened my eyes.

"What did you see?"

"That I'm not really free," I said. "Something is still tying me down."

"No. Look more closely."

I closed my eyes one more time.

"Not something," Alan said. "Some*one*. You."

"I am the one who must let go," I said.

"It is time both to let go and to be released," Alan said. "What brought you to me was your need for change. And you *have* changed. But before you move on to the next stage, you must first let go of the wanting. You are still trying to control what is outside your control. I have told you on several occasions that everything you need is inside you. This new exercise will demonstrate that. It will release you from yourself."

"That would be nice."

"And from me."

This was it—the end I had been afraid of. I felt horribly, hopelessly sick.

"From you?"

"You are not dependent on me," Alan said. "Everything I have taught you is part of you. You always had the answers inside, and now you know how to find them. It is time to let go, and time for me to release you."

"I've been clingy, is that it?"

"You have been a most attentive and diligent student, Katrina. I thank you for that. But the time has come for you to stop trying to control everything and just *be*."

I realized that everything Alan had taught me was leading to this point. He had been preparing me for my future. A future in which I would have to fend for myself.

"This is one of the most important parts of the yoga practice," he said. "It is called *savasana*. It is a deep relaxation technique that will help you to let go completely."

———

I listened while Alan explained how *savasana* works: in the first stage, as the body relaxes and the breath becomes still, the brain switches from beta waves (present during wakefulness) to alpha waves (present during sleep). When this happens, the attention moves away from the world of the senses, and the mind goes into a state of tranquil awareness.

Yogis call this *yoga nidra*, "the sleepless sleep." It has the remarkable property of inducing alpha waves while the person is still awake. And then, after a time, a third type of brain waves—theta waves, which occur in dream sleep—becomes dominant.

In this state between wakefulness and sleep (similar to hypnosis, yet requiring no guidance from an outside source), it is possible to let go of what is in the unconscious mind without needing to react to it, interpret it, or respond in any way. Finally, the brain makes one more transition, to delta waves, the brain pattern of deep sleep.

It is when you are awake in deep sleep that you are able to experience pure consciousness—a state of joy, well-being, and connectedness to all things. Because of this, *savasana* has amazing psychic healing powers.

Alan asked me to lie down on my back with my knees bent and my feet flat on the floor. He directed me to draw my tailbone toward my heels in order to lengthen my lower back and had me extend my legs along the floor, keeping my pelvis in a neutral position. Then he asked me to imagine a line drawn down the center of my body, and to adjust my position so that the right and left halves felt symmetrical. I allowed my legs and my feet to go limp. Next, Alan told me to draw my shoulders down and away from my ears, and extend my arms outward into a downward V, with my hands coming to rest about six inches away from my hips, palms facing upward.

"Now," he said, "release all tension in your hands and let your fingers rest apart. Move your head slightly forward and back and then from side to side until it feels comfortable and your neck is relaxed and unstrained. Close your eyes and feel your eyelids resting gently against your eyes like flower petals."

"This is so comfortable," I said. "I feel as if I could stay here forever."

"Then you are in the correct position. Your body is now perfectly balanced. Remember this feeling."

Alan asked me simply to follow his voice as he led me toward deep relaxation. The deeper we went, the more I realized that until this moment I had never really been totally free from tension. Or of the need to try to control what was outside my control.

"Relax your right big toe, second toe, third toe, fourth toe, and little toe, and then repeat on your left side.

"Relax your right foot and then your left foot.

"Relax your right and left legs.

"Relax your pelvis and genitals, then all of the muscles in your abdomen and lower back.

"Relax your upper torso.

"Relax your entire right palm, and then your right thumb, index finger, middle finger, ring finger, and little finger. Repeat on the left hand.

"Relax your right forearm, elbow, and upper arm, and then your left.

"Relax your shoulder girdle and neck.

"Relax your eyes and let your eyeballs sink deeply into their sockets.

"Relax your nose.

"Relax the rest of your face and your jaw.

"Relax your lips, allowing them to separate slightly.

"Relax your tongue and feel the roof of your mouth soft and lifted.

"Take up to twenty steady, even breaths, gradually increasing the length of the inhalations and exhalations."

I counted out the breaths one by one until I no longer knew

when one stopped or the next one started. I was filling up the air around me at the same time as it filled me up.

I was becoming the breath.

Then Alan told me to release any thoughts of breathing and to desist from all effort.

"And now let go of everything that is still holding you back."

My limbs felt soft and heavy, my breath was low and quiet, and my thoughts continued to slow down until they were no longer thoughts but clouds that floated far above me. My head was emptied of everything. Even the ambient sounds—traffic in the street, a class in the studio next door, the distant rumble of the subway far below—were fading away into nothingness.

And then, a minute or two later, time slowed down. No, more than that. Time ceased. There was no time. There was . . . nothing.

Blackness. Emptiness. Nothingness.

And then time had started up again and it was accelerating faster and faster—

And I was no longer on earth, in New York, in the yoga studio, lying on the floor.

I felt as if my body were separating itself into a billion particles that were being blown away by the winds of time—I no longer had a body at all. I was nothing but pure essence, simply floating in space, observing and being observed, without needing to impose myself on events, without letting anything affect me, without wanting—

I was somewhere in deep dark space, and all around me were the glittering points of light made by a multitude of stars and distant planets.

Glowing spirals of light and energy surrounded me, dancing around me, advancing and retreating, changing in shape and size from moment to moment. I was enveloped in bliss. And then at the bottom of my spine I felt a soft pulse, a warm, surging wave of power that slowly swept up through my spine until it reached my neck and then up through my neck to my skull, all the time growing stronger and more palpable until at last it reached the crown of my head.

Again and again it surged up my spine like a throbbing pulse—and with each pulse I felt a deeper connection with everything everywhere eternally.

And then it was as if the top of my head opened and rings of pure radiance streamed out at an incredible speed, and my whole body was dematerializing again and I was following the light into space, scattering among the stars, to become part of the Infinite—

"Katrina? Katrina—"

As if a great bell had tolled, the void around me seemed to collapse and turn itself inside out, and I was falling backward through time and space—

"Katrina? Come back now. Slowly start to deepen your breathing."

It was Alan. The sound of his voice was a beacon lighting my way home.

"Gently start to move your fingers and toes. Bring your awareness back to your body. Do not open your eyes. Rest quietly."

After a little while I became more alert. I could feel my limbs again. I had returned to earth. I had returned to my body.

"Slowly roll over into the fetal position, on your right side."

And then I understood . . .

I was being reborn.

"When you are ready, bring yourself back up to a seated position, still with your eyes closed."

Which I did, eventually. And there I sat for several minutes, without moving. Gradually my body resumed its habitual sense of place, and I became aware of the room, of Alan, of myself.

I opened my eyes.

After a few more moments of collecting myself, I said, "I've never experienced anything like that. It was . . . quite indescribable. I'll have to try to write down what happened. It sounds too impossible to say out loud."

"You crossed over into the state of deep sleep while you were still awake," he said. "You experienced *samadhi*, which is the ultimate state of pure consciousness. *Sama* in Sanskrit means 'same,' and *dhi* means 'intelligence'; in *samadhi* you experience the sameness of yourself and the Unlimited Intelligence. You become one."

"I felt so full of joy, Al, so full of well-being—as if I was connected to all things."

"Every time you practice *savasana* will be different. You might not have the same intensity of experience. This is not an exercise, remember. You must not compete with yourself to do better. On the contrary, you must let go of all wanting and needing. Everything that has brought you to this place. Then you can better understand what I have to say now, which is this: *You have nothing more to seek, because there is nothing that you need to find.*"

Alan and I sat facing each other. We were both silent.

"And now," he said, "I must prepare myself for the Thanksgiving meditation."

"Thank you, Alan. Thank you—"

"No more thanks to me, Katrina. Give thanks now to yourself for being who you are. And give thanks for everything that has happened in your life. It was all meant to be. It was all for a purpose and all part of your journey—the suffering and the pain, as well as the joy and the love. The world is a beautiful place, Katrina. I invite you to live in it with all your heart."

I could feel myself becoming emotional. I turned quickly, picked up my things, and gently closed the door behind me.

Outside, the teachers were gathering for the meditation. When I felt composed again, I went over to Charlie. We hugged.

"I hope you have a wonderful trip," I said. "I'm going to miss you."

"Oh, don't worry," Charlie said. "I'll still be here."

"I thought you were going to India."

"I am—but my astral body will visit you from time to time," she said.

I smiled. "You're very special," I said to her.

"So are you, Katrina. By the time I return, you'll be a teacher. Use your new role to spread the message of Universal Love."

"I will, Charlie, I will."

But I won't be promoting the raw food diet.

Then the doors to the studio were opened, and inside there were many colored balloons suspended from the walls and ceiling, and orange and white crepe paper was draped across the raised platform on which Alan would lead the class. The only light, shimmering softly, came from candles. The smell of burning incense filled the room. It was very festive. Immediately the mood became festive, too.

We all took our mats and sat down to wait for Alan's arrival. Soon after, the doors opened once more and he walked in and took his place at the front of the class.

"Happy Thanksgiving, everyone. This is a time to give thanks, not only to others but to ourselves as well. It is easy to forget that each of us plays an important role in life, and that if even one of us was not here, the world would not be the same. I owe you all my thanks, too, for allowing me to teach and guide you. With your desire to learn, you have helped me become the person I have always wanted to be. We are all seekers, and the miracle of the Universe is that one day, not so distant from now, we may come to understand that everything we ever wanted or needed, everything that was great in our hearts—joy and love and kindness and truth and understanding—was here inside us all the time, waiting quietly for us to discover it. Peace to you all, to all things, for all time."

We bowed our heads, and I felt tears fall from my eyes. When I looked up again, my tears making the candlelight sparkle before my eyes, I saw that Alan was smiling at me. I smiled back with all my heart.

It was time for me to find my own way.

And I was ready.

Breath Focus 12: RELEASE

Time: 15–20 minutes

Props (optional): bolster, pillow, or eye pad

1. Lie down on your back with your knees bent and your feet flat on the floor. Draw your tailbone toward your heels to find length in your lower back. If your back feels sensitive, you can slide a bolster or pillow underneath your knees. Otherwise, extend your legs along the floor. You may like to cover up with a blanket or employ an eye pad; both will help to relax you and deepen the experience. (Set a timer for fifteen to twenty minutes if you are worried you might miss your next appointment!)

2. Imagine that a line divides you down the center, and that the right and left halves of your body are evenly distributed on either side of it. With your knees about a foot apart, allow your feet to drop out to the sides. Adjust your pelvis so that your hip bones are level, and position your rib cage so that your spine settles onto the floor.

3. Draw your shoulder blades lightly together and your shoulders down, away from your ears. Place your hands, palms facing up, six to eight inches away from your hips so that your arms extend out in a downward V. Let your fingers be relaxed and slightly curled. Rest the back of your head on the floor, or place it on a blanket or pillow. Move your head slightly forward and back and then from side to side until it feels comfortable and your neck is relaxed and unstrained. Close your eyes and feel your eyelids resting gently like flower petals.

4. To scan through the various sectors of your body, first bring

your awareness to your feet. Relax your right big toe, second toe, third toe, fourth toe, and little toe. Repeat with your left toes. Relax your right foot and then your left foot. Relax your right leg and left leg.

5. Relax your pelvis and genitals.

6. Relax all of the muscles in your abdomen and lower back.

7. Relax your upper torso.

8. Relax your right palm, and then your right thumb, index finger, middle finger, ring finger, and little finger. Repeat with the left hand.

9. Relax your right forearm, elbow, and upper arm, and then your left.

10. Relax your shoulder girdle and neck.

11. Relax your eyes and let your eyeballs sink deeply into their sockets. Relax your nose.

12. Relax the rest of your face and your jaw. Relax your lips, allowing them to separate slightly.

13. Relax your tongue and feel the roof of your mouth soft and lifted.

14. Take up to twenty steady, even breaths, gradually increasing the length of the inhalations and exhalations. Then completely let go. Release any controlled breathing and allow your body to sink even farther into the floor.

15. If you find there are thoughts or memories bubbling up, try to be a detached observer, without reacting to them. Soon your mind will be completely free.

16. Stay in *savasana* for fifteen to twenty minutes. Continue to move deeper and deeper into relaxation.

17. To come out of *savasana*, gently wiggle your fingers and

toes, and deepen your breathing. Roll over onto your right side and spend ten to twenty breaths in the fetal position before slowly sitting back up with your eyes closed. Use the support of your arms to raise your body without tensing your neck and back. Let your head come up last.

18. Sit cross-legged for a few minutes to absorb the effects of the practice. And then, when you are ready, drop your chin to your chest, open your eyes, and gaze at a point on the floor as you gradually bring your awareness back to the room.

A Note from Katrina

The beauty of *savasana* is that it requires nothing from us except surrender. After all our striving to find the truth, this technique reminds us that sooner or later we must stop trying to control events and just trust ourselves enough to see what happens next. There comes a point in all our lives when the right thing to do is relax and let go. Remember Alan's words: *You have nothing more to seek, because there is nothing that you need to find.*

This pose will help you to seal Alan's teachings inside.

For someone who has not done this before, it is sometimes difficult to relax the body, usually because the mind continues to cling to thoughts and feelings. But if you stay with it, the mind grows calm, and your awareness of the outside world will gradually diminish, leaving you with a feeling of weightlessness. You might hear sounds, but they won't disturb you, and everything that encroaches on your peace will drift farther and farther away. Eventually you will let go of your need to impose yourself on the moment. When this happens you may, as I did that memorable time in Alan's room, have a profound experience of energy moving through your body. Do not feel disappointed if it does not happen the first time; there will be many more. And each time may feel different.

Practice every day, if you can. Some days you will find that you are able to go much deeper than others. If you practice consistently, before long you will not want a day to pass without experiencing this extraordinary technique, which achieves such remarkable results without your having to do anything but *let go*.

One last thing . . .

Of the many lessons to be learned from Yoga Master Alan Finger, perhaps the most important is that you do not need to move to a new city to transform yourself—or even have a Yoga Master as your personal guide. Wherever you are, you can find your truth and live the life you have always wanted, because, as Alan has often said, everything you need is already inside of you.

There will always be challenges in our lives, but once we are on the right path, these become less of a struggle and more of a pleasure.

Good luck on your journey, wherever it may lead you. I hope that one day we will meet again.

Namaste.

Katrina

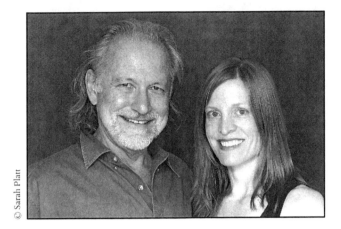

Katrina Repka has been a yoga student for fifteen years and a teacher for eight. She is currently living and teaching in London.

www.katrinarepka.com

Alan Finger has been practicing and teaching yoga for more than forty years. With his father he created ISHTA yoga, a style that is now taught in studios around the world. Although he has been a personal teacher and guide to numerous celebrities, he continues to teach regular public classes, most recently at the new ISHTA studio in downtown New York. He has been called the Supreme Yogi.

www.ishtayoga.com